The Medical Entrepreneur's
HANDBOOK

A Physician's Guide to
Income-Producing Medical Ventures

Edited by

Harvey E. Knoernschild, M.D., M.Med.Sci., FACS

CE/Q Publishers, Inc.
San Jose, California

This book is intended to offer guidance on matters
relating to the formation and operation of medical
ventures. It is sold with the understanding that the
authors and publisher are not herein engaged in
rendering legal, tax, accounting, or other professional
services. This book should not be used as a substitute
for consultations with professional advisers.

ISBN: 0-9627044-0-7

Editorial and Production Coordinator: Avram Goldstein
Cover Design: Barbara Oertli
First Printing, September 1990
Printed in the United States of America

Published by CE/Q Publishers, Inc.
58 N. 13th St.
San Jose, CA 95112
408-298-1080

Distributed by William Kaufmann, Inc.
95 First St.
Los Altos, CA 94022

Contents

American medicine is in the midst of a massive restructuring brought on by rising costs and the inability of traditional institutions to respond effectively. Unusual opportunities await the innovative medical entrepreneur who can find ways to provide high-quality health care at lower costs.

As barriers to competition are removed, physicians should develop locally needed medical facilities. Physicians can enhance their influence over health care systems, stimulate beneficial competition, and create new cost-containment methods. This medical entrepreneur, who has developed one of the nation's most successful and cost-effective surgical facilities, discusses the advantages of physician-owned facilities and debunks myths that surround them.

A free-standing urgicenter provides acute care during extended hours in a convenient location at lower cost than a hospital emergency room. This physician, who developed a major urgicenter, tells how it was done and why patients appreciate the prompt service and personalized care.

A career in occupational medicine offers the qualified physician a chance to influence workers' health while delivering a variety of fascinating related services. With proper planning, the occupational medicine entrepreneur can build an active practice within a hospital environment or in an independent facility.

In some areas nearly 60 percent of surgery is performed in ambulatory surgery centers because patients and physicians find them to be convenient and less costly. But one outpatient surgery partnership discovered that hiring a nearby hospital to manage the facility threatened its very survival.

Conflict with a hospital "partner-to-be" led this medical entrepreneur to develop a surgicenter according to his own convictions. After several years of success, a partial buyout proved the wisdom of his ways.

Because breast cancer is one of the most prevalent and feared malignancies, careful instruction in self-examination and screening mammography are in great demand. Providing these services within a dedicated facility offers women thorough education and diagnosis at a lowered cost.

High-acuity patients are being cared for at home for half the cost of hospitalization and in a more comfortable and convenient environment. Such "alternative" care systems will be the traditional systems of tomorrow. This entrepreneur's program, enthusiastically used by patients and physicians throughout California, is a prototype for the future.

Contents

Chapter 8

The InfusiCenter Clinic

Paul Scholtes, M.S., M.S., J.D., and Julia Sherman, B.S. (Pharm.)

Cancer patients who require extended chemotherapy need supervised infusion but not hospitalization. The InfusiCenter Clinic uses innovative protocols to reduce costs and treatment times in an outpatient setting that meets patients' needs.

Chapter 9

Developing and Managing an Imaging Center

Cesar Mayo, M.D.

New diagnostic imaging modalities performed on an outpatient basis have replaced many expensive and painful invasive tests. Financed by a physician limited partnership, this imaging center offers lower costs because of its reduced overhead. Patients suffer less anxiety and receive improved care in a convenient setting.

Chapter 10

Starting a Multispecialty Clinic

Peter Crandall, M.D.

The rapid rise in managed care contracting has stimulated new forms of medical practice. This physician tells how a multispecialty group, with good management and attention to individual preferences, can offer physicians a cooperative working environment and professional security during the turbulent 1990s.

Chapter 11

Recovery Care Centers

Tony Carr, B.A., M.S.

A major challenge to medicine is admitting patients to the appropriate level of care for the shortest time. The recovery care concept offers a new kind of facility for surgical patients who do not need the complex and expensive technology of an acute care hospital. By keeping patients for shorter stays and avoiding cost shifting, the recovery care center provides high-quality care at a significantly lower cost.

Chapter 12

Marvin Rawitch, M.D.

The "inter-indemnity trust" concept developed by these physicians offers "pay-as-you-go" coverage to more than 3,500 physicians. With careful selection, aggressive risk management, and quality control by members, this innovative insurance program brings the cost of professional liability coverage far below the premiums charged by traditional insurers. The program has improved patient care and reduced physician overhead.

Chapter 13

Harvey Knoernschild, M.D., M.Med.Sci.

Many physicians know that joining a PPO/EPO group can benefit their practices and reduce health costs in their communities. During the 1990s, the successful provider groups will deliver high quality care in the most efficient manner. This physician discusses the evolution and advantages of PPO/EPOs and offers insights on how physicians can develop their own groups to control the high cost of health care.

Chapter 14

William Sueksdorf, M.D.

Utilization review has generally failed to lower health care costs because it usually avoids direct peer-to-peer contact. This company uses local physicians to communicate cost-effective use of resources directly to their peers. With the rapid growth of managed health care, this innovative approach can be adapted to existing utilization review programs.

Chapter 15

Paul Schrupp, B.A.

The impetus for physicians to develop a new medical facility often begins when their hospital becomes more committed to creating new programs than to improving existing services. This experienced adviser outlines how a medical entrepreneur can plan, design, and finance a free-standing facility that will provide superior patient services.

Preface

During the past decade, the American medical system has been overwhelmed by unprecedented changes driven predominantly by spiraling costs. Barely a day passes in which we don't read or hear about the high cost of health care, whether expressed as a percentage of the gross national product or as an industry-specific inflation rate which compares poorly with the consumer price index. Resonant voices from all sectors of society, including medicine itself, are calling for a nationalized health system, and they will get their wish if the current delivery system fails to achieve lowered costs. It is time for action!

Society is forcing the health care system into competition—competition among physicians, among hospitals, and among entire health care systems. And it's no surprise. Competitive dynamics in a free enterprise system will result in lower costs and in better products. However, the traditional health care institutions so far have failed to respond to this need to reduce costs. Rather than improve internal efficiency, they continue to raise prices and increase the cost to consumers. They have thus relinquished any claim to special legislative protection or economic privileges. It is now up to individual physicians and other concerned providers to respond to this challenge and join the search for solutions. Albert Einstein once said, "The significant problems we face cannot be solved at the same level of thinking we were at when we created them."

It is certain that every provider and medical group has been, or soon will be, affected by the increased competition generated by the consumers who make up the marketplace. Many providers already feel caught up in a maelstrom of change, one in which they have lost control of their own destiny. The way physicians practiced years ago has virtually disappeared. The personal satisfaction of simply caring for our patients has been diminished by the modern concerns of copayments and reimbursement rates. Some physicians are resentful of these changes; others are confused and bewildered; most don't understand them or even want to. Physicians wish to be left alone to practice medicine in one-to-one relationships with their patients. They long to be immune from the nuisance and interference of the outside world.

Unfortunately, becoming a medical hermit doesn't work. The strength of the marketplace is far greater than the wishful thinking of providers who don't want to get involved. The marketplace has stated very emphatically: "Give us superior, cost-effective health care under the existing system or we will replace it with a nationalized system." With each increase in health insurance premiums, the forces pushing us toward a nationalized health care system get stronger. The threat is very real, and if we want to preserve the free enterprise fee-for-service method of payment, time is growing short.

Despite the pressures, we should not be forced to apologize for wanting to preserve our capitalistic reimbursement system. It has helped to create the world's best health care system, even if it costs too much. Recently, we watched the crumbling of command economies and the revival of free enterprise in the nations of Eastern Europe. We have observed, once again, that when the incentive for individual initiative is thwarted, inefficiency and slothfulness can result. Rather than move into a nationalized delivery system devoid of initiative or reward for innovation, we should make the existing system cost-effective and thereby more accessible.

There is a brighter side. For the provider who has kept current with the needs of the market, these dynamic changes in medicine bring dramatic opportunities to be creative and innovative, to become entrepreneurial leaders within the community, and to directly reduce patient costs. If we replicate these actions in thousands of communities, we professionals can rein in the rising cost of health care.

Former U.S. Surgeon General C. Everett Koop has challenged the private sector of medicine to solve the health care system's problems, saying that the industry's own solutions would be preferable to government intervention. "More government involvement isn't desirable, and it probably won't work," he said. "But unless the private health care sector gives us some alternatives, it will have only itself to blame for what happens."

This book describes some of the creative projects that now exist in the health care field. There are, after all, numerous ways to develop innovative, alternative medical services that will meet the needs of patients, payers, and providers. The experiences shared by these authors should stimulate individual readers to examine their own hidden talents and professional goals and objectives. Some will be encouraged to become entrepreneurial leaders and assume an active role in meeting the needs of the marketplace. By developing alternative medical projects and ventures, they can help provide the superior cost-effective health care the marketplace demands.

The Medical Entrepreneur's Handbook was written to encourage health professionals to discover and use their entrepreneurial and innovative talents. Each author has taken an alternative concept through the initial planning and development and into the operational phases. The result in every case has been an innovative way to improve the efficiency and quality of care.

This is a "How I did it, and how you can do it, too!" book. Each project is fully described, including the perceived reason for its development, the response it received from hospitals and other providers, how it has been cost-effective, and how the quality of patient care has been improved.

The Medical Entrepreneur's Handbook is a resource for health care professionals, financial advisers, and medical facility developers.

Harvey E. Knoernschild
March 15, 1990

Introduction

The Industrial Revolution of Medicine

Medicine in America today is undergoing the most dramatic change since the advent of health insurance and third-party payments. The driving forces are the exceptionally rapid increase in the cost of health care and the system's failure to respond in any effective or meaningful way. It is impossible to fix the blame on any one involved party, so all aspects of the health care system should be reviewed and adjustments made where necessary.

In many respects, the nature of the current upheaval in medicine is very similar to the Industrial Revolution of 150 years ago. The changes now affecting the practice of medicine are a product of technological advancements, an oversupply of manpower, and gross inefficiencies within the existing delivery system. With these similarities, it is appropriate to label this period of change as the "Industrial Revolution of Medicine." All the players in the current revolution—the hospitals, payers, patients, and providers—now are coming to grips with serious internal decisions. How should each respond to these external demands for increased efficiency without compromising the quality of care? What can government do to encourage competition and eliminate protectionist regulations?

Since the time of Hippocrates, the personal relationship between doctor and patient has always been considered above mere financial considerations. Needed services often were rendered without payment. Sometimes payment was made with chickens or an exchange of services. This pragmatic but effective barter system was replaced by health insurance and a "third-party administrator." With the multiple and complex reactions caused by positioning this entity, the payer, between the patient and the physician, each side has shrunk away from bearing personal responsibility for the cost of care.

There are many causes for the high cost of health care. People continue to abuse their bodies through neglect and poor personal habits, and the consequences of their preventable behavior account for nearly 50 percent of health care expenses. Their expectations of cures and perfect outcomes have led to costly defensive diagnostic testing and unnecessary procedures. New technologies for the diagnosis and treatment of diseases have developed rapidly, much faster than physician knowledge of their appropriate utilization. When communication between patient and physician deteriorates, malpractice suits are filed, forcing tremendous increases in medical overhead. Hospitals have had the luxury of unchecked price increases and the ability to shift unpaid costs to private payers. For many years, insurance companies did nothing to control unnecessary and inappropriate claims. They simply relied on premium increases year after year to cover their burgeoning payouts. These and many other factors have driven health care costs upward and helped produce the current crisis in the system.

It is quite revealing to examine the dilemmas facing each segment of the health care industry in the current chaos. Most are reluctant to make the changes necessary to reduce the cost of care within their own market areas. Hospitals, for example, have had a monopoly on caring for the sick and postsurgical patients for centuries. But now they see more than half of their former surgical patients choose the outpatient or ambulatory setting. How should the hospital respond? Does the hospital start its own surgical center and compete with the members of its medical staff who pioneered ambulatory surgery in the community, or does it purchase an interest in an existing facility? What about home health care? Today, some patients with serious medical problems are being discharged from hospitals very early and being well cared for at home by high-acuity nursing programs, and at a significant savings. Should the hospital develop its own vertically integrated delivery system? Can the medical staff be made to use the new programs? Can the hospital administration manage the new program with greater efficiency than it manages itself at present? As these innovative programs force the hospital to lower charges, should hospital associations promote legislation to thwart competition and cost-effective alternatives? After all, if the healthy patient who pays full price for half price service is drawn to an alternative facility, hospital profitability will dwindle. But why should the payer for the healthy patient subsidize the hospital? Shouldn't the patient pay only for the true cost of services used?

Hospitals are burdened with the inefficiencies of inflexibility and bureaucratic overload. Most have had to assume the costs of a market development department and a physician services director, each of whom raise costs while contributing nothing to health care. Hospitals also suffer from "cost shifting," whereby a portion of the cost of caring for patients in underfunded government programs is shifted to private-payer patients. As innovative health care projects start in their neighborhoods, hospitals accuse them of "skimming the cream"—the sought-after revenue from the profitable healthy patient. Rather than looking internally for ways to become more cost-efficient, hospitals resist competition and change. But because hospitals were built for a different time and a different way of doing things, are they becoming institutional dinosaurs? Why should hospitals be granted preferential tax treatment as non-profit institutions while other health care facilities are not?

The nation's entire labor force is being buffeted by these changes. Under new benefit plans, workers are expected to assume more of the cost of health care through copayments and higher deductibles. The employee is given a limited list of providers from which to select a physician. The long-time family doctor has been replaced by a more efficient clinic physician who is willing to discount fees but cannot afford to take the time to sit and chat. The patient worries about whether he or she chose the right doctor and whether there will be too much or too little care. The patient must now make sure the physician obtains proper authorization from an impartial review organization before any expensive diagnostic or therapeutic procedures are performed. Failure to get approval may cost the patient dearly. Health care has become complex for the patient who wants high quality and affordable care delivered in a warm and personal manner.

Employers, Taft-Hartley trusts, and other private payers have been swept along by this Industrial Revolution of Medicine. After seeing their costs continue to skyrocket, they are reinforcing the call for real competition in the health care delivery system. By offering exclusive contracts to groups of physicians and selected hospitals, they are winning significant discounts for services. But after these contracts have been negotiated, how does the payer maintain access to the more economical alternative programs and non-traditional facilities which are not forced to shift costs? A healthy employee who needs a hysterectomy or cholecystectomy could have it performed in an ambulatory surgery center with the post-surgical care given in a recovery care center at significant savings over traditional hospital care. Should payers be forced to send all their beneficiaries to contracted hospitals, or will they choose to maintain access to any alternative facility which can provide appropriate and superior cost-effective care? Employers are walking a tightrope, trying to keep employees happy with their benefit packages while finding ways to reduce their insurance premiums.

Government-mandated health care programs have been grossly underfunded and have shifted part of the cost of care for the poor and elderly onto the backs of non-government payers. Employers and other private payers are subsidizing these mandated governmental programs. In their effort to prevent erosion of the hospital's private-patient base, some legislators find it necessary to restrict and hobble worthwhile innovations. Is the government's answer to the marketplace one of protecting the status quo despite inefficiencies and higher costs? Instead, shouldn't government be encouraging the development of new cost-effective programs and allowing them to compete with traditional institutions on a level playing field?

This medical revolution is now fully under way, and it is causing many providers great anxiety. Will they be able to continue practicing what they consider to be high-quality care, or will they be forced to follow protocols that don't permit individualized variations? Providers are worried about a declining patient base, shrinking personal income, and rising overhead costs, especially for professional liability insurance. They are being forced to focus on these issues and to make crucial decisions for their future. Should they abandon solo practice and join a multispecialty group? Should they join a preferred provider or exclusive provider group to market their services and increase their access to patients? How much can a provider discount fees before there is no profit left?

Time is running out for the American fee-for-service system, which has led the world in medical care for more than 75 years. It is about to be abandoned to the whims and antics of health care planners and economists, most of whom have never cared for a patient. As physicians, nurses, and other health professionals ponder the future, we must evaluate our individual talents and seek opportunities within our own communities. We must stop and ask ourselves some vital questions:

• What are the goals and objectives for the remainder of my professional career?

• How can I continue to provide high-quality patient care while practicing in a more cost-effective manner?

• What alternative health care programs have been successful elsewhere and could be useful in my community?

• Where can I be most effective in making health care services more affordable to my patients?

I believe the nation's medical community is a sleeping giant waiting to be awakened and stimulated into action. The key is to apply this giant's greatest untapped resource—the entrepreneurial spirit many physicians and other providers have kept deep inside. They must be encouraged to respond to this dynamic and challenging marketplace. As health care professionals, we have spent our entire careers learning to understand and respond to patient needs. We have probably observed numerous ways to reduce costs without sacrificing the quality of the outcome.

Already many physicians across the country have developed alternative facilities with tightly controlled costs and patient charges substantially lower than those in hospitals. We are the natural advocates of patients, and that must continue. As such, we must become active in developing innovative ways to provide superior, cost-effective care. If those who know the needs of the patient and have the motivation to be creative don't take the leadership role, who else might step in? Who will do it with the patients' interests foremost?

The Medical Entrepreneur's Handbook is intended to challenge providers to develop novel medical projects and ventures that will provide the type of health care the marketplace demands. If we act together, we *can* have a major impact on the nation's response to skyrocketing health costs and see to it that first-rate patient care isn't sacrificed in the process.

1

Should Physicians
Own Medical Facilities?

Alan H. Pierrot, M.D.

There is substantial evidence that Americans are unhappy with their health care system. Recent polls indicate more than 70 percent of the population would prefer a national system such as Canada's. Escalating costs have everyone—patients, providers, insurers, and payers—concerned. A complex variety of solutions has been proposed. Physicians have tremendous potential to offer constructive solutions to our health care problems, but in the past, our society has not established an environment that encouraged physician solutions. But times are changing, and physicians should keep pace by unlocking their dormant entrepreneurial instincts to make constructive contributions.

An important factor in the escalation of health costs has been the lack of true competition in the health care marketplace. The consumer is frequently not sophisticated enough or does not have access to the information necessary to make a well-reasoned purchase of health services. Because he cannot make a price-versus-quality judgment, his purchase is not price sensitive. Providers are then not rewarded for offering a superior product at lower cost, so they do not. Competition does not develop, and prices remain high. This environment must change if we are to slow health care inflation.

A number of states are attempting to stimulate competition by removing barriers to competition, such as the certificate of need process. Physicians should enter this increasingly price-sensitive, competitive marketplace and develop products such as surgery centers, imaging centers, laboratories, birthing centers, cardiac catheterization labs, fitness centers, cancer treatment centers, HMOs, and even hospitals. Physicians are better qualified for this role than they may think. They know the patient, his disease, and his needs in and out of the hospital better than most others on the health care team. They are the best judges of quality of care and therefore best able to assure it. They are intelligent, innovative professionals who are likely to envision new solutions if the environment permits their implementation.

There are many compelling reasons for physicians to invest in local health delivery systems:

Diminishing fee-for-service income. Physician income will inevitably drop. In 1995, the number of trained physicians in the United States will be nearly double the number in 1975, and this increased supply comes as patients are making fewer office visits and consumers are organizing to obtain discounts. If physicians are to maintain present income levels, they must find alternate income sources. Those sources are available in health care, but in the past physicians have ignored them and the profits have gone to others.

Access to management. Physician ownership of a health service business such as a surgery center provides investing physicians with prompt access to management. They can wield far more influence over the service than in the average hospital. Decision-making in hospitals is slow and cumbersome, and physicians usually are not given enough information to exercise much influence. A physician in a hospital has less impact on management than a physician as an owner of a health care facility.

Profit. Well-run health facilities with high utilization (not to be confused with unnecessary utilization) can be profitable. For example, in Fresno, California, 96 physicians founded the Fresno Surgery Center/Recovery Care Center. They created the finest outpatient surgery center in their community, one that within four years was in the top five percent nationally for volume. In less than three years the center has been profitable enough to pay substantial dividends to the original physician investors. The value of the original shares more than doubled.

Larger surgery centers need 2,500 to 3,000 cases annually to be profitable. Thirty surgeons who do 100 outpatient cases a year can form a partnership, perform their surgery in their own facility, and reach break-even in the first year. Certainly such a program would be far safer for the physician owners than investing in the weird schemes that all too often are attractive to doctors.

Safety. Risk is diminished by broad physician participation. We have little ability to affect an oil-drilling project, but we can certainly see to the success of a surgery center, clinical laboratory, or imaging center. Twenty internists who establish a quality lab with fair fees can almost be assured a first-year profit. The same concept applies to surgeons and a surgery center, or neurosurgeons and neurologists for a magnetic resonance imaging unit, or urologists and a lithotripter, or obstetricians and a birthing center. All that is required is physician leadership. When physicians create and invest in a facility, that facility then has a strong referral base and a high enough volume to compete on price. And when the price is low and the quality high, there is no conflict of interest for the physician investors. Indeed, such a formula works to the community's benefit.

Timing. The timing is right. In California the certificate of need requirement was abandoned in 1987 in hopes of stimulating competition. At least 10 other states do not have CON laws. Physicians should now begin to look for niches in the marketplace where they can provide more efficient services through health care boutiques that take a service and provide it more personally, more efficiently, and less expensively than hospitals. That is hardly a conflict of interest for the physician owners.

Community service. The availability to consumers of choices other than hospitals for the same service creates healthy competition that keeps everyone on their toes, improves perceptions of health care costs, and lowers actual costs. For example, when the Fresno Surgery Center/Recovery Care Center opened in December, 1984, one of the large local hospitals reduced its outpatient surgery charges by 30 percent. It is doubtful that those charges would have been rolled back without the physician-owned Fresno Surgery Center/Recovery Care Center.

Pride of ownership. A nice feeling goes with owning a quality facility. A number of physician investors have expressed that to me, and I feel it too.

Knowledge leads to innovation. The physician owners of the Fresno Surgery Center/Recovery Care Center began by gathering information about the economics of an outpatient surgery facility. They saw the advantages of increasing volume as they recognized that many of their patients did not require the full range of expensive inpatient services. This led the partnership in 1986 to successfully sponsor innovative legislation permitting ambulatory surgery centers to keep post-operative patients for up to three nights in recovery care centers. The Fresno Surgery Center/Recovery Care Center built the first such 20-bed unit in an annex to its present building. This has increased the volume in the surgery center and permitted us to reduce charges dramatically (by as much as 50 percent for some procedures) for patients healthy enough to enjoy the recovery care facilities. This exciting legislation was the result of a physician partnership and physician innovation.

The health care boutiques can be organized in any manner that makes sense to the local physicians. In Fresno we have had good luck with limited partnerships, but there have also been successful hospital-physician joint ventures. Anything that is fair is likely to work if there is strong leadership, substantial local physician support, adequate capitalization, and a good end product at a reasonable price.

If you establish a physician owned entity in your community, be prepared for a variety of objections and misconceptions about the investment.

Vocal individuals, physicians, and lay people will contend that it is unethical and a conflict of interest for physicians to own shares in a health care facility to which they refer patients. In California in 1985, these critics introduced legislation, subsequently defeated, to make physician ownership and utilization illegal. Congress has considered similar legislation. At first glance, this viewpoint has validity. But it does not hold up under analysis. For example, the average profit for The Fresno Surgery Center/Recovery Care Center in 1987 was $160 a case. The average physician owned slightly more than two of the partnership's 220 shares. Thus the average surgeon-investor who brought a case to the center made $160 divided 110 ways, or $1.45. The conflict of interest comes into play when a surgeon recommends an operation to a patient (the higher the fee, the greater the conflict)—not by where the surgeon actually performs the surgery. If he operates in the center, he will make another $1.45 more than he would make by performing the same procedure in a hospital—hardly a conflict. Physicians deal with far greater conflicts everyday: the surgeon who recommends an operation that he will perform, the cardiologist who recommends cardiac catheterization that he will perform, the radiologist who recommends an angiogram—these are the conflict of interest areas in medicine, not physician ownership of health care facilities. If the procedure is indicated and the price fair, there is no conflict, and a fair price is more likely in a competitive setting than in the monopolistic tyranny of the certificate of need process.

The hospital view is that physician boutiques skim the cream— the private patients—and leave hospitals with indigent patients and money-losing services that a community needs but does not fund adequately. This argument is flawed because it assumes that only hospitals are entitled to profit centers (a particular irony in the case of not-for-profit hospitals) and that forcing them to compete is somehow a blow against the community. If that argument is accepted, non-hospital innovation will die because the profitable services will be off-limits to entrepreneurs. I've tried the same logic with other orthopedists, telling them they could only compete for my non-paying patients, but, alas, no luck. I've also tried it with a local hospital that is operating a sports medicine facility and skimming patients from me. Again, no luck. The challenge for physicians is to develop the competing entities, and the challenge for the hospitals is to figure a way to compete—not hide behind the skimming argument. The need to provide indigent care is not an acceptable rationale for overcharging and underserving private patients.

Critics also fear that competition will develop between rival physician groups. That should not be a problem. Physicians are already competing with one another for patients, and that will only increase in the future. My purpose is not to suggest physician monopolies, but to stimulate physicians to form their own local health care businesses that will survive only by offering superb service at a fair price. Competition between local physicians will only raise the level of care for everyone.

Another objection is that many physicians are not good businessman. But most communities have a number of physicians with the interests and ability to organize a physician-owned business. They can then run the business (more and more doctors are going into management) or hire competent administrators.

One valid concern is that physicians are not team players. This is a major hurdle. Some physicians will never organize a partnership and will resent those who do. They are the second-guessers who will not invest initially because the project is "too risky" and who later use hindsight to rate a successful entity as a "sure thing." Others are too conservative in their investment approach and will not risk capital in a start-up. Because the goal is a broad base of physician support, both types must somehow be included. They must be shown the tremendous potential for both community service and profit.

Many fear that physician investment will guarantee success. This is absolutely not true. In my experience, physicians will always choose quality of care over profitability. To their credit, physicians would rather lose their investment than support a facility that does not deliver superb care at a competitive price. Even that does not guarantee support. The Fresno Surgery Center/Recovery Care Center offers both superb care and competitive pricing, yet some investing physicians use the facility for less than half of their outpatient cases.

Some will view physician involvement in the marketplace as greed. This corollary to the skimming argument is the result of the simplistic tendency to view not-for-profit organizations as good, pure, and altruistic and for-profit entities as greedy and interested only in the bottom line. But both types of organization are community-oriented and worried about the bottom line and their self-preservation. Some not-for-profits have gone so far as to establish for-profit subsidiaries. A recent extensive study of both types of health care facilities concluded that for-profit entities actually returned more to their communities than not-for-profits. When The Fresno Surgery Center/Recovery Care Center sponsored legislation to establish recovery care centers, the heaviest opposition came from local not-for-profit hospitals. Here was a for-profit physician entity attempting to implement a less costly alternative clashing with not-for-profit hospitals. Physician greed is not the issue, and physicians should not be put off by that claim.

Most of the forces in medicine today have the side-effect of limiting physician influence in the marketplace, and the traditional physician position has been to avoid the marketplace. But physicians should go beyond the half-truths and establish physician-controlled boutiques that deliver superb care at a reasonable price and generate a profit. Physicians will enhance their influence over local health care systems, stimulate healthy competition, and gain insights into cost containment that office-based practitioners cannot appreciate—all while earning a profit. It has worked in Fresno. How about your community?

ALAN H. PIERROT, M.D., received his education from the University of Michigan and Stanford University (A.B. 1964, M.D. 1966). He interned at University of Colorado Medical Center, then served two years active duty with the U.S. Air Force. Following a residency in orthopedics at University of Kentucky Medical Center, Lexington, he went into the private practice of orthopedics in Fresno, California. In 1984, he formed a partnership with other physicians and opened the Fresno Surgery Center. In 1988, this partnership built the first recovery care center in California. Dr. Pierrot has chaired several committees and served as president of the medical staff of Fresno Community Hospital. He is a Diplomate of the American Board of Orthopedic Surgery, and a Fellow of the American Academy of Orthopedic Surgeons and the Western Orthopedic Association. Dr. Pierrot is chairman of the Center for Competition in Healthcare and general partner of the Fresno Surgery and Recovery Care Center. He is available as a consultant in the areas of ambulatory surgery centers and recovery care facilities.

2

The Free-standing Urgent Care Center

Mark Congress, M.D.

As I donned my white coat and waited for the first patients to walk into the Cupertino Emergency and Family Medical Clinic that summer morning in 1979, I felt cautiously optimistic. The stakes were very high. Everything I had worked for since graduating from Georgetown Medical School in 1963, all my training and experience as an emergency physician, and all my possessions were on the line. To finance this project in a San Francisco Bay Area suburb, I sold my precious red Jaguar convertible and our condominium apartment in Lake Tahoe, and I put a second mortgage on our house. And I wasn't making this gamble alone. My brother Miles, also an emergency physician, and Lorraine Parish, business manager of my hospital-based emergency medical group, were coming with me.

Although free-standing emergency clinics provide acute health care in a convenient location and at a significantly lower cost than hospital emergency rooms, no one in California had yet succeeded with such a venture. In 1979, they were called "emergicenters." But because that term suggested 24-hour service and treatment of acute ambulance cases, the industry eventually dubbed them "urgent care clinics," or "urgicenters." Dr. Robert Gordon opened the first urgicenter in New Providence, Rhode Island, in 1975.

Hospitals traditionally equip and staff emergency rooms for worst-case situations—heart attacks, shootings, and automobile accidents—and staff them around the clock. This means that the patient who visits at 10 a.m. with a sore throat helps pay the overhead for the patient who presents at 4 a.m. with a drug overdose.

Urgicenters can charge substantially lower fees than hospitals because they don't have to operate food services, complex clinical laboratories, and the very latest medical technology. Nor do they maintain hundreds of employees on the payroll. That's why their average charge in 1989 was $54—less than the basic fee charged by most hospital emergency departments for merely signing in. Urgicenters stock basic life-support equipment to treat heart attacks that occur on-site, but that's the extent of preparation for truly life-threatening emergencies. Hospitals depend on emergency rooms to fill beds, but an urgicenter's success depends on efficiency and patient volume. Urgicenters cannot accept major accident victims or emergency patients, and the ambulance companies are well aware of this restriction.

According to the National Association of Freestanding Emergency Centers, at least 80 percent of patients who go to emergency rooms suffer from non-urgent conditions. They end up in the emergency room because it's the only place to go after regular physician office hours. When the hospital emergency staff is tied up with a serious injury or illness, other patients cannot be evaluated for long periods—often up to several hours. Because urgicenters don't mix severely injured accident victims with sick children, as emergency rooms do, a visit averages only about an hour.

Urgicenters stay open 12 to 16 hours a day, seven days a week. If they are conveniently located, efficient, and reasonably priced, these clinics will attract patients who prefer not to visit the hospital emergency room. I decided early in my planning that patients should not have to pay $100 or more for treatment of an after-hours sore throat when the average physician's office charge for the same service at that time was about $35.

By 1982, with medical costs rising at twice the rate of inflation, third-party payers began to recognize the cost-saving potential of these clinics. In that year, insurers and government were paying 92 percent of the nation's $278-billion annual medical bill.

I first became interested in the urgicenter concept when I read an article by Dr. Robert Gordon in Modern Healthcare magazine. Like me, Dr. Gordon was in his early forties and had spent his career practicing in hospital emergency rooms. He, too, had grown weary of the sterile hospital decor, the long lines, the antiseptic odors, the "stat" pages, and the numbing impersonality that were part of the fabric of emergency medicine.

He had phased out of his hospital-based emergency practice and rented 3,000 square feet in the first-floor corner of an office building shared by an insurance company and a dentist. Dr. Gordon's office had a waiting room, a reception desk, examining rooms, a nursing station, a small laboratory, and an x-ray room. On the front window he painted in gold letters: "Emergency Clinic Open 8 a.m. to 10 p.m."

At first, only a few curious patients showed up, but within 18 months, the word had spread: patients could drop by the emergency clinic without an appointment and receive excellent medical care at a reasonable price in an attractive setting—without waiting for hours. The clinic soon became so busy that Dr. Gordon set up another office in the nearby city of Warwick.

Dr. Gordon had found a way to offer the quality of care he knew he could provide. He didn't have to suffer through hospital board meetings or undergo a certificate of need review to try his ideas. And it wasn't like riding herd over momentary patients in the emergency room. He could follow some patients from illness or injury to healing without charging high hospital fees. Patients would fill his waiting room, he figured, because they wanted to, not because they had no alternative.

As I read about Dr. Gordon's clinic, I realized this was exactly the sort of career change I had been awaiting. After logging more than 50,000 hours in emergency rooms, I knew I needed to change direction to satisfy my own creativity and refresh my spirit. And my experience had prepared me well. I had already directed three emergency rooms, so I understood the administrative pressures. This seemed like the perfect solution.

With my curiosity piqued, I picked up the telephone in the spring of 1977 and called Dr. Gordon to arrange a visit. I wasn't the first physician to express interest in his practice, and because the doctor would be unavailable for an extended period, his secretary suggested I visit a similar operation in Austin, Texas. She wisely pointed out that the Texas clinic was a lot closer to California and somewhat newer and that this would help me appreciate the concept from the ground up. With great anticipation I made an appointment with Dr. Dennis Ela, owner of the Minor Emergency Center North in Austin. I flew to Austin and found myself standing in front of an attractive building in a strip shopping center in what could have been any modern American suburb.

I went into the simple but attractively decorated waiting room and introduced myself to the receptionist, a pleasant, neatly dressed woman who was clearly identified with a name tag on her blouse. She welcomed me, told me that Dr. Ela would be with me shortly, and asked if I would mind waiting in the lobby because all the rooms and offices were occupied. I sat down in a comfortable chair, picked up a current magazine and began to appreciate the ambience of this, the newest concept in emergency medicine.

Actually, I didn't mind waiting at all because I could observe the reactions of several patients when they handed their paperwork to the receptionist. No one objected to paying by cash, check, or credit card instead of through insurers. Several even commented on how reasonable the fee was. I watched a laborer who was injured on the job, a mother with two small children, a teen-ager who hurt his wrist in a skateboard mishap, and an elderly woman with a bad cough. Patients who were acutely ill or injured were taken to the doctor immediately, and the receptionist was careful to announce to the remaining patients that they would be called as soon as possible.

My initial impressions were favorable, and they were strengthened when Dr. Ela and his nurse graciously gave me a tour. The clinic was well-designed, the examination rooms were clean and well-equipped, and the feeling was one of a physician's private office. He handed me a copy of the floor plan and a list of necessary equipment and suggested ideas on what it took to establish a successful clinic. After spending the afternoon seeing patients with him, I walked out of the urgicenter feeling pleased by the high quality of care this type of practice could provide.

On the flight home, I jotted down the key ingredients of a successful clinic: a location in a nice neighborhood on a main thoroughfare, easy access, adequate parking, and, very important, a large lighted sign on the street. Few other physicians would be practicing in the ideal area, a good hospital would be five to 10 miles away, and a mix of residential and industrial neighborhoods would be nearby to form the patient base. I figured that a population of 35,000 or more was necessary to provide enough patients to support the clinic and that the urgicenter would need enough capital to last at least one year before turning a profit.

From my vantage point in emergency rooms in Redwood City and San Mateo, I could see that the nearby growing community of Foster City might meet my criteria. I shared the concept with my six emergency group partners. They liked the idea, and we invested $15,000 each.

The Foster City Emergency Medical Clinic opened on April 1, 1978, but the deck was stacked against us. The medical staff at Mills Hospital in San Mateo was aghast that a group of upstarts from the emergency room would compete with them for the few Foster City patients they considered within their market. This opposition put our group's emergency room contract at Mills in jeopardy. That was bad enough, but we were then unable to obtain a sign permit, making our location at one of the area's busiest intersections completely hidden from passing traffic and pedestrians. Because the venture was undercapitalized, we had no money to advertise adequately, and we remained utterly invisible to the public. After three miserable months, we couldn't pay the rent.

Despite this negative experience, months later I wanted to try again—but this time, on my own terms. I shared my ideas and concerns with my wife Lorie, who expressed her faith in me and her willingness to share the financial risk. I once worked in the emergency room of El Camino Hospital in Mountain View, and many patients there had asked why I didn't open a private practice in Sunnyvale or Cupertino, where few physicians could be found. Now, eight years later, I was curious to see if things had changed in this town 18 miles south of my home.

I turned to "physicians" in the Yellow Pages and was amazed at how many were listed in Sunnyvale—and how few practiced in Cupertino. I hadn't been to Cupertino in years, so I decided to check it out. Lorraine Parish and I drove there in less than 25 minutes, and we were pleased to find well-kept middle-class residential districts and some industrial zones. Kaiser Cement and Aluminum, Hewlett-Packard, Four Phase, and a fledgling computer company called Apple were all based in Cupertino.

Segments of the city's two main thoroughfares, De Anza and Stevens Creek boulevards, were well developed, but other sections of the roads led past apricot orchards and empty lots. At the southern end of Stevens Creek was a charming 50-year-old granary. Along the busier northern side I noted parcels with "build to suit" signs. Dr. Ela, the Austin physician, said we'd need about 4,000 feet of clinic space and parking for at least 25 cars. We called the developers of these lots and found they either were the wrong size or were already taken.

Yet I felt certain that Cupertino was the right city. All I had to do was find an appropriate location, impress a developer with the merits of the project, tap a funding source, and convince the city manager and residents of Cupertino they needed a clinic! I also had to win approval for an illuminated urgicenter sign and figure out how to capture patients without competing with neighboring physicians.

Through a real estate broker, I met Terry Rose, a successful Cupertino area developer planning a 10,000-square-foot, one-story building on the corner of Stevens Creek Boulevard and Vista Drive. He had one potential tenant, a golf professional who planned to lease 6,000 feet for a pro shop and indoor driving range. Rose was impressed with my ideas and agreed to build 4,000 feet to suit. He asked if I would mind being in the rear of the rectangular building, whose short side would be fronting on Stevens Creek Boulevard. I told him that as long as there would be a lighted sign clearly visible to street traffic, that would pose no problem. When viewed from the street, our front door would be on the side of the building. In fact, I liked the idea of having a second entrance in the rear so injured or acutely ill patients could bypass the waiting room.

We shook hands and agreed to proceed with the project with a three-year triple-net lease at about $3,500 a month. He recommended a local architect with medical design experience, and I made an appointment. As I drove home to Woodside, the commitment I had just made hit me like a ton of bricks. I wondered how I was going to finance this urgicenter. I considered physician-investors, but they would require detailed business plans and lengthy one-on-one meetings. I didn't have time for that. So I went to banks to find out about loans. They all asked the same thing: "You want to do what?" No one had heard of the urgicenter concept, and banks, being conservative institutions, were unwilling to risk the capital.

In desperation, I decided to use our home as collateral to obtain the loan. Interest rates were at a favorable 10 percent at the time, but because my home was already heavily mortgaged, the only available deal required me to pay 10 basis points up front. The $153,000 floating-rate loan allowed me to pay interest only for four years with the entire principal due as a balloon payment at the end of the term. (Remember that during the four years from 1979 to 1983, interest rates rose from 10 to 22 percent, which was hardly favorable for launching a business.) But the loan wasn't enough. I was forced to use our savings and put our condominium, our camper, and other assets up for sale. We went in with $200,000 of working capital.

Next we had to design the facility and prepare lists of needed supplies and equipment. My brother and I wanted working space for pediatrics, ophthalmology, ear, nose, and throat work, minor surgery, pelvic examinations, orthopedics (including casting), and laboratory. The x-ray department required an adjustable table, darkroom and x-ray processor. Each area had to be equipped with sinks, cabinets, and shelves.

I knew that hospital emergency room patients with even minor chest pain or shortness of breath would be wheeled directly to a "crash room" into which the doctor and nurse would disappear. Our "crash room" would be an open area directly connected to the nursing station, equipped only with curtains for privacy, so the nurse and physician could monitor the patient's EKG while remaining aware of other clinic activity.

We wanted the waiting room to be comfortable, spacious and attractive. In hospital waiting rooms, receptionists often sit behind opaque, sliding glass windows that, in effect, keep patients outside the emergency room. Our concept was to join the waiting room to the reception area so patients would not feel isolated. It would be carpeted and furnished with drapes and sturdy, comfortable furniture. Pleasant music would play in the background, and guests would see a large selection of current magazines and interesting periodicals.

The urgicenter would need space for a physician's office, storage of patient records and x-rays, a staff lounge with kitchen facilities, a bookkeeping area, and an office for Lorraine. We included a central supply area with an instrument sterilizer, a telephone, and a clinic-wide paging system. The plumbing plans were complicated because an urgicenter requires many sinks and a shower for croupy babies and victims of toxic spills. Separate restrooms were provided for waiting-room guests, patients in the examination area, and staff members.

In the hospital setting, we had grown accustomed to the luxury of picking up a telephone and requesting a respiratory therapist and a ventilator whenever necessary. But in a free-standing urgicenter, if we didn't have a ventilator and bottled oxygen and someone skilled in respiratory therapy, the patient would not receive appropriate care. This is one example of anticipating the need for special equipment. One never knew what might be needed one moment to the next, so we had to learn to do everything ourselves.

We decided each examination space would be multipurpose and identical in size, configuration, and cabinetry. Each room was outfitted with sinks, towel dispensers, blood pressure cuffs, otoscopes, ophthalmoscopes, tongue blades, percussion hammers, flashlights, Band-aids, Ace bandages—essentially everything I had ever wasted time searching for in ERs and clinics.

As I was designing cabinets, I remembered that a nurse once told me that the biggest space-wasters were drawers that didn't open all the way. So I insisted on drawer slides that pulled all the way out. This relatively minor detail added a few hundred dollars to the total cost of the project, but it has saved countless hours of physician time and allowed us to reduce the size of storage areas.

One of the most annoying causes of patient delay in hospital ERs is the unavailability of special rooms. We decided to use rolling carts to move specialized equipment around to enable any examining room to be used to apply a cast, examine an eye, suture a laceration, or stop a nosebleed.

Once the architect's working drawings were completed, Terry Rose submitted them to Cupertino officials for approval. The plans were accepted, and he went on to obtain bids from contractors.

Lorraine meanwhile was busy applying for business and operating licenses and hunting for equipment suppliers. Soon the office in my garage was filled with plans, sample books, and used equipment, and the telephone was ringing off the wall. I never expected to be consulted on such decisions as whether to buy Muppets wallpaper for the kiddie room, blanket warmers, refrigerators with ice makers, and centrifuges; whether to choose built-in water fountains or bottled water coolers; or which colors to select of tiles, doors, baseboards, carpets, and drapes, but I was. I bought a small pickup truck and soon was roving the Bay Area to pick up gurneys, defibrillators, surgical carts, and sterilizers. Everything went into my garage for storage.

Early one morning in May, 1979, I drove past the corner of Stevens Creek and Vista boulevards on my way to meet Terry Rose. I had been there several days before and was frustrated to see that nothing had been happening on the vacant property. But this time, a construction shack with an attached power line had magically appeared. I let out such a loud whoop of joy from behind the wheel that I frightened a pedestrian! Finally, my dream was on its way! I met the construction foreman, and from that day on I visited the site almost every day. I didn't know the first thing about reading a blueprint, but I was curious enough to learn.

The contractor said construction would take about 90 days, giving us ample time to plan the delivery of supplies, hire the staff, order telephones, place Yellow Page ads, and attend to myriad other details. We set up a "Coming Soon" sign that displayed the telephone number of the garage/office in my home. The response was incredible. Many people called to say they were delighted to have a clinic in their neighborhood. Some wanted to know what an emergency clinic was, and others were looking for jobs or trying to sell us supplies. Lorraine handled each call with care and diplomacy.

She also observed the construction whenever possible. One day while poking around the site, she noticed that no one had run the drain line for the x-ray processor—a timely observation. Fortunately, the construction supervisor had no trouble adding the pipe at that time. Later, when the walls were framed and the sheet rock was about to go up, I noticed that soundproofing was missing from between the walls of the examination rooms. Again the timing was right, and the contractor remedied the problem without tearing out walls. I had many other things to do, but watching the building take shape was exciting and useful, so I took a few minutes each day to drop by.

Several months earlier, Miles and I had brought our families to visit our parents in New Jersey. During our stay, we had dinner with a cousin who was a marketing director for Safeway supermarkets, and we shared our marketing ideas with him. He gave us a most valuable piece of advice: Contact the director of the local chamber of commerce. When I returned to California, Lorraine and I made an appointment to have lunch with Frank Mulkern, director of the Cupertino Chamber of Commerce.

Mulkern could not have been more pleased when we told him our plan. He had long dreamed of seeing Cupertino become self-sufficient, with its own public transportation system, post office, library, shopping centers, senior citizens center, and hospital. Our plan came in the midst of the gasoline crisis of 1979, and Mulkern thought Cupertino residents should be able to obtain any merchandise or service without having to drive beyond the city limits. He already had scored a major victory with his support of a new cinema complex in the Oaks Shopping Center, and the prospect of improving health care in town fired him up again.

Years earlier, Cupertino tried to encourage construction of a hospital, but the multi-city hospital district chose to build in a neighboring town instead. Mulkern thought the urgicenter would fill the gap in acute care, so he gave me the names and telephone numbers of dozens of merchants, educators, business people, and service club members who would want to learn about the clinic. He suggested contacts at Kaiser Cement, Kaiser Aluminum, Apple Computer, Hewlett-Packard, Motorola, De Anza College, and the city government.

After the urgicenter construction plans were approved, I spent six days a week for almost three months campaigning across Cupertino, meeting people and telling them about the clinic. One meeting often led to another, and soon I found myself telling the same jokes and making the same speeches to groups at breakfast, lunch, and dinner meetings. I was timid at first, but one warm reception followed another, and before long I began to enjoy myself. I had never been able to sell anything to anyone before, but I was so enthusiastic about this concept that I couldn't find enough hours in the day to promote it.

I knew I would need input and support from my fellow physicians, and I did not want any of them to perceive the clinic as a threat. Only a handful of primary care physicians practiced in the urgicenter area, and most seemed to be cordial and receptive. I told them we would operate 105 hours a week, including weekends and holidays, and that we'd be happy to cover their practices during their off hours. We had no intention of stealing their patients. We promised that after treatment we always would send patients back to their primary physicians with a copy of our record of the visit.

One physician, a pediatric allergist, told me Cupertino was absolutely the worst possible location for an emergency clinic and that he was moving out of the area precisely because of the dearth of patients. He complained that there weren't enough multispecialty clinicians, the patient population was unstable, and patients preferred large group practices near El Camino Hospital in neighboring Mountain View. And if that weren't enough, he warned me that the Rexall Pharmacy on busy De Anza Boulevard was going out of business. I felt a few butterflies in my stomach as he offered this depressing litany, but I knew I would have to press on.

I sent announcements to most members of the Santa Clara County Medical Society and followed up with visits or phone calls to many of them. I told them I would be referring patients to them for consults and hospitalization, and I asked them to send their business cards to me when the clinic opened if they were interested in working with us. I told Nielsen Buchanan, administrator at El Camino Hospital, that one reason I chose Cupertino was to be able to refer patients to his hospital. He welcomed me, and we began a professional relationship that continues to this day.

While I was getting to know the physicians and potential sources of patients in Cupertino, Lorraine was advertising for receptionists, nurses, and x-ray technicians. Because we were to be open two shifts a day, seven days a week, we would need three full-time equivalents for each position. First we sought a head nurse who could help us hire the rest of the nursing staff and stock the clinic.

Our bank in Cupertino let us use its conference room for interviews, and our very first applicant was a capable, personable, experienced nurse who lived around the corner from the site. Jeanne Schlick has been our head nurse ever since. She reviewed and revised our purchasing lists and joined Lorraine in the office, which was overflowing with strange-looking items. Her first job was to finalize the "crash cart" for cardiac patients, and she found that a Sears Craftsman tool chest mounted on casters worked fine. She screened other nursing applicants and arranged for me to meet one at the incomplete clinic building.

When I met Donna Brandt in the parking lot, my impression was that she was competent and pleasant, so I hired her, handed her a hard-hat and brought her in to the construction site to show her around. Leaning on the half-finished nursing station counter in the flickering light of generator-driven lamps, I told her about the concept of free-standing emergency clinics and rashly predicted we would see up to 100 patients a day. I must have seemed overenthusiastic at the time, but it turned out to be a conservative prediction. Our one-day record is more than 200 patients!

As the building neared completion, last-minute details demanded attention. My wife volunteered to wallpaper the patient rooms. No one knew much about hanging cubicle curtains, so I ended up on a ladder with a drill, molly screws, and a screwdriver. That was useful, because it pointed out our need for tools, a ladder, and a vacuum cleaner to clean up the mess I always made. I told Lorraine and Jeanne that I was going shopping, and they gave me a list of items to pick up at K mart. I'll never forget the expression of the cashier when I pushed up to the counter with hammers, screwdrivers, assorted screws and nails, 15 coat hooks and door stops, note pads, toilet paper, light bulbs, a dozen current magazines, a toilet plunger, three radios, a guest register, two coffee pots, six baby bottles, children's toys, boxes of diapers in three sizes, and two sizes of sanitary napkins. I wonder what she thought I was doing.

Finally, the wallpaper and curtains were hung, the waiting room carpeting, drapes and furniture had arrived, the financing was complete, and the city of Cupertino had given its blessing to our project. My wife suggested a family vacation. She knew that once the clinic opened, I would be there day and night until it was a success. Also, our oldest child, Deborah, was heading off to the University of Colorado early in September, and I hadn't seen much of her all summer.

My wife arranged for us to spend a week on a houseboat on Lake Shasta with our three children and some friends. It turned out to be a wonderful trip, and we were surprised by a visit from an old friend who lived in nearby McCloud. I was telling him about the clinic when I suddenly remembered that it was Thursday, the day the city sign committee was due to consider our application for a lighted sign. I knew that Terry Rose and Lorraine Parish would represent me, and there should be no problem. But I felt uneasy, and the more I thought about the meeting, the more I believed I should be there. I remembered my experience in Foster City with the clinic that wasn't visible because it had no lighted sign.

We boated to the dock where our car was parked, and I drove to Redding to catch a flight to San Francisco. Lorraine picked me up and took me with her to the meeting. When it came to the clinic, the board asked for me in person. As I answered their questions, it became clear to me that they felt it unnecessary for a "doctor's office" to have an illuminated sign. I tried to remain calm and deliberate as I pointed out the special purpose and need for this clinic. I emphasized the fact that most people in an emergency situation have difficulty remembering how to drive and would certainly have trouble trying to find a building that was not clearly labeled as an urgicenter and visible from the street.

The committee responded favorably and approved the sign. I flew back to Redding feeling relieved that I had gone to the meeting. I learned long ago to trust my instinct, particularly with a critically ill or injured patient. This was just another example of how the same instinct applied to a different set of problems.

When the vacation ended, I returned to Cupertino with renewed vigor and beheld a completed building. The sign had been ordered, the staff was on board, and most of the supplies had been delivered. Only a few days before the Labor Day weekend of 1979, I learned that it took several weeks after completion of a building before it could be occupied. That wouldn't be soon enough for our plans, so I made an appointment with the city manager. Fortunately, I had already met him in my travels, and I explained that we were ready to open and had announced that to the public. He was kind enough to allow us to cut the waiting period for a certificate of occupancy to only a few days, and we knew we could open on September 4, 1979, the day following Labor Day. We spent that entire weekend doing last-minute unpacking and cleaning and reviewing staff protocols.

The afternoon before opening day, Linda Guidero, a longtime Cupertino resident, and her teen-age son Robert visited the office. He had injured his elbow in a football game and wanted to be our very first patient. I explained that our permit was not in effect until the next morning, but examined the youngster to determine if he needed immediate treatment.

The examination showed a possible fracture of the head of the radius in his elbow. I advised the mother that a sling would make him comfortable for the night. X-rays were indicated to see how long immobilization would be required and how soon he could play football again. She thanked me, and they went home, only to return before 8 a.m. the next day to make sure Robert was our first patient.

After months of hard work and anxiety, the opening was almost anticlimactic. I treated Robert Guidero and gave his family a tour of our facility. Mrs. Guidero told me that she had nine children, all of them athletic, and all of whom had friends who played sports. The Guideros are a wonderful family, and they have proven to be a source of many patient referrals.

Anticipating long, slow days, I had brought my journals, my saxophone, and an exercise bicycle to the clinic to pass time. But as it turned out, there were always things to do. Many people whom I had met before we opened came for tours. Each new patient took a tour and walked out with a brochure. Our growth was far more rapid than anticipated, and soon the days were flying by.

I trained the staff to assist me in calling patients at home to see how they were doing. When I had worked in emergency rooms, I kept a list of patients I was concerned about and called them during my shift. Good news or bad, it was important to me to know the status of patients I had seen. Most were grateful for the call, some were frightened, and some expressed dissatisfaction. I learned a lot about patient care from these calls and knew I should continue this practice at the urgicenter.

Shortly after we opened, the Cupertino city manager dropped by with good news. The Medevac Ambulance Company had won the advanced life support contract for Santa Clara County, and it chose Cupertino as its paramedic operations center. Cupertino was delighted, but the only available housing was at the nearby city-owned yard, which had a few bunks and a kitchen. Medevac units work in 24-hour shifts, during which the paramedics often get dirty and need to shower. Our clinic was a logical choice for their base—especially because we expected some of our patients would require paramedic transport and we had the needed shower facilities. With Medevac on hand, we'd save a lot of waiting time.

As a token of his gratitude for our having solved his problem, the city manager asked me if the city could do anything for me. I told him I had read about cities that placed highly visible reflector signs along the streets to direct patients to emergency clinics. If I would provide the signs and choose existing signposts to mount them on, he said, the city would provide the manpower to hang them. Within two weeks, seven reflecting signs on main roads directed traffic to the clinic.

When the news of Medevac's involvement with our clinic was printed in the Cupertino Courier, a group of angry residents living in apartments behind the clinic protested to the city council. They were concerned about the noise of ambulance sirens around the clinic, not to mention the certain death and disease that would be visited upon their backyards.

I pointed out to our neighbors that ambulances would not be delivering patients to the clinic and that it functioned essentially as a physician's office with extended hours and emergency capabilities. Ambulances transporting patients from the clinic to the hospital would not use their sirens until they were on Stevens Creek Boulevard. Because we were closed from 11 p.m. to 8 a.m., there would be no overnight activity. And it was a lot quieter than the sirens wailing from the existing firehouse on the corner across the street from us at any hour of the day or night. Medevac officials made a similar case, offering charts and graphs with statistics on ambulance noise. I could tell from the audience response that we were not very persuasive.

Then Ed Cali from the granary asked to speak. He got up in front of the citizens of Cupertino, most of whom were his customers and contemporaries, and recalled how one of his workers had fallen from a high scaffold a few months earlier. When they called for an ambulance, it took almost an hour to arrive because of heavy traffic. He said he had suffered along with his man for what seemed like forever until the ambulance got there. "You people ought to be grateful that this clinic is in Cupertino," he scolded. When he was finished, the crowd burst into applause and the board unanimously approved Medevac's clinic location.

During the first two months, our patient volume grew slowly but steadily as patients spread the word. We aided that process by tailoring our services to the needs of our community. We are in constant contact with our clients, and we quickly respond to their problems and requests. Many patients and potential patients called for medical advice, and we developed a protocol for handling them. A local firm asked if we could provide physical therapy for one of their workers with a back problem. We said yes and obtained a traction therapy table, a hot-pack unit and an ultrasound machine. We set it up in a room which also housed our lab (consisting of a centrifuge and a microscope at that time) and thus began our PT department. We taught the nurses how to perform ultrasound treatments, apply hot packs and provide cervical traction. From these humble beginnings, we now have a full-time department with complete equipment and three technicians.

If the school districts ask us to help immunize students, we do it. If they need someone to speak at career day, I am happy to appear. We have developed computerized instructions for each employer to ensure that they are notified of the status of every worker we treat. We process on-the-job injury reports as quickly as possible. Serving our community this way accounts at least in part for our success.

During our third month, we started to get busy. At times I could barely keep up with the volume, and the pace started to take its toll. I had been typing all my charts and trying to finish them immediately after each patient visit to avoid falling behind. One night I sat down at midnight confronted by 75 charts to type before I could go to sleep. To make things worse, I had another 15 hour shift starting at 8 a.m. the following day.

Miles was having the same problems keeping up, so we decided it was time to start looking for another practitioner to relieve us during peak periods. But we never knew in advance when it would be busy. We figured that a family practitioner would be a logical second person to have on staff. I called Dr. William Fowkes, the director of the San Jose Medical Center family practice residency program and made an appointment to see him. After I told him what type of practice we had and what I felt our needs were, he suggested we not hire another physician and instead get a PA. I didn't know what a PA was, so he explained that physicians' assistants complete an accelerated curriculum at reputable medical schools and provide limited medical treatment under the supervision of a licensed physician.

I was skeptical when I telephoned the California Association of Physicians' Assistants. Within an hour, I received a call from Nick Perrotto, a certified physician's assistant and arranged an interview. When I gave him my standard emergency doc screening quiz, which many MDs have failed, he passed with flying colors. Nick has been with us ever since.

Over the years, we have received a great deal of local and national publicity. Stories about our innovations appeared in the Cupertino Courier, the San Jose Mercury News, USA Today, the San Jose Business Journal, South Bay Today, Modern Healthcare, and Ambulatory Care, a newsletter for the National Association of Freestanding Ambulatory Clinics. Shortly after we opened, KPIX-TV in San Francisco aired a series about our clinic. We have been extremely fortunate to have been so well-received by the citizens of Silicon Valley.

Over the years the Cupertino Emergency and Family Medical Clinic has changed with the community. We have expanded twice and now occupy the entire 10,000-square-foot building. The clinic offers physical therapy, orthopedics, and internal medicine services as well as urgent care. Our original staff of six now totals 45. My brother Miles and Lorraine opened an unrelated clinic in Los Altos that is nearly identical to our original effort. They are doing very well.

My urgicenter became an affiliate of El Camino Hospital and changed its name to Cupertino Medical Clinic. El Camino purchased an equal partnership interest in the management corporation that runs the clinic, and I own the professional corporation that provides the medical services. Where once we looked out our windows at apricot orchards, now we see a huge, modern town center with two nine-story buildings under construction for Apple Computer.

Our clinic once was the only one in the area. I counted 22 in the Santa Clara County 1989 Yellow Pages. Yet we still see more than 100 patients a day, and 40 to 50 of them are new to the clinic even after all these years. Many of our old patients come back, having tried one or more of the newer clinics in their neighborhoods. Most tell us that the attitude of caring they found at the Cupertino Medical Clinic cannot be reproduced. I will do my best to see that this tradition continues.

MARK I. CONGRESS, M.D., received his undergraduate education from Rutgers University (A.B. 1959) and his medical training at Georgetown University School of Medicine (M.D. 1963). He served a rotating internship at Milwaukee County General Hospital, Milwaukee, Wisconsin. He entered the United States Navy and served three years as flight surgeon in Vietnam, Okinawa, and Cherry Point, North Carolina. Dr. Congress practiced emergency medicine in the San Francisco Bay Area for eight years during which he was chairman of the emergency departments of three different hospitals. In September, 1979, he founded and became medical director of the Cupertino Medical Clinic, where he currently practices. He is a charter member of the American College of Emergency Physicians and has been active in his community on the Disaster Preparedness Committee and the Drug/Alcohol Abuse Council. Dr. Congress is available as a consultant in the area of urgent care centers.

3

Developing the Occupational Medical Clinic

Lester Sacks, M.D., Ph.D., and Claire Sacks, R.N., B.S.

An occupational medicine practice offers qualified physicians a chance to broaden their understanding of their patients' lives and to shape the health of workers while delivering a variety of fascinating related services. A typical employee spends more than eight hours a day on the job performing tasks in an environment with which most physicians are not familiar. Indeed, the beauty of occupational medicine is that the practitioner has an opportunity to live patients' lives with them—to understand what they do, how they do it, and the impact of work on their lifestyles. This role demands a familiarity not only with primary care skills, but toxicology, ergonomics, workplace psychology, and preventive care. It also offers an excellent opportunity for the aggressive physician to secure contracts as a corporate medical director and eventually enhance the growth of his or her primary care practice by retaining employees as private patients.

With proper planning, the occupational medicine entrepreneur can build a thriving practice within a hospital or in an independent facility. We will examine the advantages and disadvantages of each format based on proposals involving occupational medicine specialists and various Southern California hospitals as well as my own survey of independent occupational medicine practitioners.

The first step in determining whether you should launch an occupational medicine practice is to write a business plan. Decide where you are, where you want to go, and the time frame necessary to achieve these goals. Do your homework. Understand the community. If you're going to limit your practice to an occupational health service, make sure you understand where the employers are and what industries they represent. If the employer base is consistent and unlikely to change, this could be a self-limiting opportunity. A static environment is acceptable if that condition is evaluated as part of the business plan. If the area has multiple forms of industry and is undergoing expansion, there is greater potential for practice growth. Each industry should be analyzed separately.

When planning an office, you must decide what you are trying to achieve and whether you will be limiting yourself in the future if you fulfill the plan. Whether hospital-based or free-standing, the facility should be planned so you can grow and so that it lies within reasonable distance of your home. Unless you have multiple facilities and a large organization, you must be able to serve clients and patients 24 hours a day. If a physician employee doesn't show up, you must be present. Someone has to be available to cover fully any service you are marketing.

With a free-standing facility, the most important concern in determining a location is whether the community is still growing or is built-out, and whether the area has existing medical competition. If there is none, it might be prudent to expect competition to develop as the industry grows. Because medical care is a service business, you must identify the level of service the competition has developed and maintained. If there is competition, you must at least match the others' level of service. However, the most logical way to offset the effect of competition is to be creative and develop new services.

Assuming the area is appropriate, you must then consider the location of the facility vis-à-vis your own home. How close is the free-standing facility to the bulk of the industry being served? What barriers to patient accessibility exist, such as railroad tracks, heavy traffic, inadequate public transportation, or limited parking? Is there street parking? Building parking? If you have selected a large medical building, must patients and clients pay parking fees? Are there enough spaces to serve everyone?

When the time comes to market the practice, an active chamber of commerce can be extremely helpful. Find out if other organizations in the community will allow you to become a member to facilitate marketing your service. Make sure that medical essentials such as ambulance service, materials management services, and telephone answering services are available. It is vital that you interact successfully with businesses, workers, and other physicians. You must develop activities that make you visible and marketable to the community.

No occupational medicine specialist works in a vacuum. Every other medical specialty can legitimately claim to have some interest in the so-called occupational health arena. Orthopedists, neurosurgeons, dermatologists, ophthalmologists, pulmonologists, and family practitioners all are independently working in that arena, so an occupational medicine provider is likely to be perceived initially as a threat. It is imperative that the entrepreneur make amends, in a sense, with the community and not allow an adversarial situation to evolve. Think of these other physicians as resources that you must understand and use, and they will understand that you are also a resource to them.

When considering competition, you must assume that physicians practicing in the same community have evaluated it as you have. Whenever a new facility is developed in a medical community, the overall level of service and quality of care does improve to meet the competition. If you are the only game in town, clients must take what you offer, which means you might overlook service to some. With competition, the employer will expect more intense service.

There is no point in developing an adversarial relationship with competitors. It has been my experience that it is best to know your competitors' strengths and weaknesses so you can offer employers the menu of services you are best equipped to provide. For example, if you have surveyed the community and found that your competition does not provide extended office hours and the employers have three shifts, it would behoove you to extend your hours. Dealing with your competition can only help you fill the gaps in their service and identify your facility as different and of high quality.

Most of your competitors are likely to be close to the industrial area. You must locate the practice within three miles of the employer. It should not take more than 12 minutes for an injured worker to reach the office. Of course, this may change depending on whether you are in a metropolitan area or a small town, but these general parameters are useful. Only if you are developing a hospital-based occupational medical center will the distance in travel time or miles become less important, because most people define the hospital community in much broader terms.

Raising the money to start an occupational medicine enterprise may be the least enjoyable aspect of this process, but rest assured that the resources are out there. In formulating a capitalization plan, you must examine the free-standing occupational medicine center and the hospital-based practice. Banks, venture capitalists, and hospital and medical suppliers are more than willing to address your financial needs. Review more than one method with your accountant to find the solution that best fits your situation. Young entrepreneur physicians often fail to see the entire financial picture. Many say, "I don't need a whole lot of money. I can generate it as I work." Philosophically, this seems fine, but it simply doesn't work! The physician will be a day late and a dollar short most of the time. Undercapitalization is the most common cause of financial disaster in a medical practice or any other enterprise.

In the financial world, you can be extremely creative, but you should know the basics about some conventional methods of financing a medical practice. The community bank can lend money if you have written a business plan with income and expense projections. You can glean this information by talking to competitors and surveying the medical community. Without an appropriate short-term and long-term business plan, you will have trouble winning a line of credit. It is not uncommon for the bank to offer a three to five-year note with smaller payments in the beginning and heavier payments toward the end of the term. If you proceed with this method, make certain you are prepared to refinance at the end of the period. Do not expect to receive a long-term note with a low interest rate. It simply isn't profitable for commercial banks to charge only a few percentage points above the prime rate.

Commercial banks will offer two types of notes. The most common procedure is to divide the total loan principal and interest charges into equal monthly payments. The bank might issue a series of short-term (six months to a year) personal notes with interest only due until a balloon payment is payable upon renewal of the note. The overall cost of the second method is appreciably less than the long-term method, but that benefit comes at higher risk. You could have your note called or you may not be able to refinance it at the anticipated rate. Or worse, if your credit rating declines, the bank is less likely to renew the note. Obtaining the money to finance your enterprise is one thing, but generating sufficient income to repay the loan is quite another. Approach this conservatively. You always have an opportunity to pay more overhead, but you will not often have an opportunity to pay less.

The entrepreneur may also consider dealing with venture capitalists. The problem with venture capitalists is that they charge a higher interest rate and request a substantial percentage of the profit. A venture capital corporation will require you to become its partner. Unless you are going to open a very large free-standing medical facility with tremendous income potential that requires substantial financial resources, a free-standing or office-type occupational medical practice is best run without venture capitalists.

Another financing option is to create a partnership with other physicians willing to help you capitalize the venture. They may act much the same as venture capitalists, except they would agree to service the facility to allow for increased hours of operation and a referral system that might benefit their other practices.

The most common way to approach a new community is to purchase an existing practice. The practices of physicians who have died, retired, or decided to spend less time in a certain location are frequently available. A medical practice broker known to the local physician community or one who advertises in medical journals can help the purchaser find going concerns. In determining a fair value for the practice, the buyer must consider whether it is strictly a workers' compensation practice with little or no private patient care. If so, the practice will generally sell for 75 to 100 percent of the gross annual revenue. But make sure the numbers make sense. Figure out how many patients the physician would have to see to achieve the figure. As a general rule, you can use a $50 to $60 charge per visit in a workers compensation practice. If we were to assume a charge of $50 per visit, a practice with annual gross collections of $500,000 in seeing 10,000 patient visits for the year. That number divided by 12 months and 22 1/2 workdays per month (assuming no weekend hours) means an average of 37 patients per day.

Does the price include the valuable accounts receivable? Good receivables give you a direct line of cash. If you bought the practice for $400,000 and the good receivables are about $150,000, you can finance the receivables for at least 70 or 80 percent of their face value. This puts you in a position to capitalize yourself and pay the current owner of the practice a significant down payment. Accounts receivable financing can be difficult because you are literally using money needed for the general operation of a facility, but if you have no alternative for developing cash resources, the accounts receivable provide an option for a cash purchase. The receivables coming in each day would already be spoken for, and you could not touch that money, but you are also continuously creating new business. It is a delicate balance.

If the numbers are accurate, the practice seems to have growth potential, and you choose to buy it, you must find out by what method the physician or heirs wish to sell it. Does the current physician have a good reputation? Does he or she wish to maintain a relationship with the facility? What are the financial needs of the retiring physician? After you have addressed these questions, you can talk about terms.

In the final analysis, I prefer a free-standing occupational medicine facility that has developed a contractual relationship with a hospital. This alliance can place many significant resources at your disposal and help build the practice rapidly. Services at the hospital would be limited to educational programs, such as cardiopulmonary resuscitation and first-aid training, and psychiatric and substance abuse activities. That would give the physician time to practice medicine and interact with employer-clients. I would also educate and perform related services with staff emergency physicians to expand the occupational medicine practitioner's on-call coverage.

With a hospital-based facility, there is no need to deal with banks, venture capitalists, or physicians' widows, although a hospital-based occupational medicine center resembles a venture capital project or a partnership. In a joint venture, the hospital will provide the space, the equipment, and additional capital. A hospital can produce a much broader range of programs to support the practice than an individual physician could manage. Hospitals of all sizes usually have specialists on the payroll to manage community planning and education and maintain emergency rooms, x-ray departments, laboratories, physical therapy units, and rehabilitation services. Together, they create a better image for the practice and permit the occupational medicine specialist to provide a wider range of appropriate care.

The primary disadvantage of a hospital-based practice is that physician income expectations are appreciably lower than outside the hospital. But a hospital-based operation can give you crucial financial support and insulate you from personal financial risk. Hospitals are in the business of making money, so you and a reputable attorney should carefully review the proposed terms and conditions. Nonetheless, if you spot an opportunity to enter into a hospital-based medical facility arrangement instead of a free-standing practice, consider the hospital plan carefully.

Occupational medicine services rendered by either the free-standing clinic or the hospital-based center are similar. They include clinical services (caring for work-related injuries and on-the-job illness, conducting pre-employment examinations, disability reviews, and physical therapy); wellness programs (lifestyle factors in health risk assessment, preventive care, cost containment, productivity advice); employee assistance programs (job-related stress, substance abuse, and productivity issues); and environmental health programs (industrial hygienics and technical review of the workplace).

At Level One in primary services, the occupational medicine specialist in a free-standing facility would:

• Perform physicals for executives, job applicants, injured workers planning to return to the job, and workers whose health status must meet government regulations, such as pilots and others in transportation industries.

• Diagnose, treat, and evaluate work injuries.

• Evaluate and rate injuries for workers' compensation claims.

• Provide on-site advice, such as hazard assessments, and fill corporate medical directorships (a format only for individual practitioners).

A Level Two practice would also reside in a free-standing facility and be structured to provide Level One services plus:

• Perform audiometric, pulmonary, and cardiovascular testing.

• Conduct screening and follow-up examinations and health risk assessments.

• Offer health education, such as breast cancer information.

• Help companies develop in-house substance abuse policies and employee assistance plan referrals.

• Set up educational programs to prevent accidents and develop awareness of alcohol and drug use. Such programs can be physician-directed or handled by an educator from most hospital units.

• Provide rehabilitation services, including physical therapy, back injury education, and pain-control programs.

Level Three services deal with injury prevention and physical fitness, and while all can be performed in a free-standing facility, most can be more effectively and inexpensively handled by hospital educators. These include on-site exercise programs, stress testing, and medical self-care programs, such as talks on nutrition and use of medications, as well as informal and formal luncheons with specific topics. This level includes psychological counseling programs on subjects such as smoking cessation and time management. Stress management programs include relaxation and biofeedback clinics.

While the occupational health services rendered by a health care facility and a hospital-based occupational center appear to be identical, the hospital provides emergency room care and is adept at many services that are difficult for independent private practices to provide. With some services, such as industrial hygienics and technical review of the workplace, there is no difference, because most practitioners in either setting would hire a subcontractor for these services. Additional costs for the operation of the hospital facility are somewhat reduced because allied services and ancillary departments, such as x-ray and physical therapy, are more directly available through the hospital. The drawback is that services rendered by the hospital are more time-consuming and expensive.

Don't expect the hospital-based occupational facility to have the backing of the physician community. As a general rule, most physicians view it as an irritant and perceive this joint venture as a hospital scheme to compete directly with them. It has been my experience that a specialist, such as a cardiologist, becomes threatened by a hospital joint venture with an occupational medicine practitioner even though there is little or no competitive activity. That's just the way it is. A community's private practitioners feel that the hospital is taking away their bread and butter even though they handle little or no worker's compensation or occupational medicine. It takes a concerted internal public relations and marketing effort by the hospital and the physician to reduce anxiety. If successful, that effort will result in harmonious and productive relationships.

One of the most important benefits of a hospital-based venture is its heightened appeal to the employer community. When marketing a service to a populous industrial community, a hospital will find it easier than an individual practitioner to achieve goals because the hospital has a physical presence and an established reputation. If the hospital is a good one, employers will think that everything the hospital does is appropriate. Because of the superior personnel and financial resources at the hospital's disposal, client education is probably the most significant area of difference between an independent practice and a hospital-based arrangement. They have the resources on their payroll to do this. At a free-standing facility, you do not. You will have to contract these services out, and that means you might not be familiar with them or be able to assess the quality of programs your clients are receiving.

This is why it is appropriate in the business plan to target the joint venture between a hospital and your free-standing facility. It can be a very workable arrangement. Find out what the hospital is doing currently, what the hospital would like to do, and where you might fit into the scheme of things. See if you can provide the hospital with a new service without competing directly with the institution.

The skill you possess as a physician is what makes you an entrepreneur, and hospitals do not necessarily want to be entrepreneurs. Indeed, they prefer to avoid this image, but it certainly is acceptable for a physician to be an entrepreneur.

LESTER SACKS, M.D., received his undergraduate education at George Washington University (A.A.) and Long Island University (B.S.). He earned a medical degree (D.O.) at the College of Osteopathic Physicians and Surgeons, Los Angeles, in 1956, and his M.D. degree in 1962 at the California College of Medicine, University of California, Irvine. He interned at Parkview Hospital and received his residency training in general preventive medicine at the University of California, Los Angeles. He took his M.P.H. degree at UCLA and in 1982 received his Ph.D. in Oriental studies from the College of Oriental Studies in Los Angeles. He is board certified in both family practice and occupational medicine and has practiced these disciplines for more than 30 years. He serves as medical consultant to many corporations and is senior vice president of medical affairs for Beech Street of California (a managed health care company). He has written and lectured widely in the area of occupational medicine. He is president of the Western Occupational Medical Association (1990) and chairman of the private practitioners' section of the American College of Occupational Medicine.

CLAIRE SACKS, R.N., B.S., received her degrees at Mercy Hospital School of Nursing and the Sacred Heart College in North Carolina. She has taken postgraduate education at the University of California, Los Angeles, the University of California, Irvine, and at the University of Texas. She has been a medical administrator for the Medical Clinic of Torrance and assistant operations officer for a multi-clinic network. She also has been an independent consultant in practice management.

Lester and Claire Sacks are available for consultation in the field of practice management.

4

The Care and Nurturing of an Ambulatory Surgery Center

Alex Fraser, M. D.

The idea for our free-standing ambulatory surgery center in Escondido, California, originated in 1983 with the anesthesiologists who practiced at the community's only hospital, Palomar Medical Center. We believed that such a facility would be more convenient for patients and physicians, and would cost the patients less. Many physician partners expected an outpatient surgery center to bring us greater independence, relieve the pressures of being on call and caring for emergency patients, and provide a second source of income. We believed that an outpatient surgery center would allow us to provide more personal care in less intimidating surroundings. Starting times would be more reliable, physicians would be burdened with less paperwork, and bureaucratic interference would be minimized. The advantages seemed overwhelming, and so we decided to proceed.

On March 3, 1986, we opened the Escondido Surgery Center two blocks from the 318-bed hospital and 11 miles from the nearest other surgery center. The $4.1-million center now draws 75 percent of the outpatient surgery in Escondido—an outflow that has cost Palomar $2 million a year. Remarkably, in spite of the loss, the hospital has not significantly changed its outpatient surgery program.

The surgery center has 100 staff physicians, virtually all of whom also practice at the hospital. Many of the original free-standing surgery centers, such as the one started by Dr. Wallace Reed in Phoenix, Arizona, in the late 1960s, were owned and operated by anesthesiologists. But we determined that our chances for success would improve if we invited our surgical colleagues to become full partners.

We began the organization in 1983 by inviting all Escondido physicians to a planning meeting. Although we faced immediate skepticism about the project and most of the guests chose not to participate, a core group of physicians understood that it was a sensible proposal. As the project got under way, several gastroenterologists and the radiology group at the hospital asked to be included so they could perform outpatient endoscopy and radiology procedures in the free-standing facility. We ultimately attracted 30 physician partners from a broad cross-section of medical specialties, including anesthesiology, general surgery, otolaryngology, ophthalmology, orthopedics, plastic surgery, gastroenterology, radiology, and gynecology.

We believed we needed to establish the project quickly to get the jump on competition and retain local control. Only later did we learn that a proprietary chain was considering developing a surgery center in Escondido until it found that we local physicians had our own enterprise under way. The local hospital was in an expansion phase, and although it was replacing outmoded operating rooms, the surgery department there would never be able to handle the entire load of inpatient, outpatient, and trauma patients who would descend on the hospital if it established an outpatient unit. The administration was preoccupied with the expansion plan and unable to help us ward off out-of-town competition. The hospital administration failed to recognize potential consumer demand for free-standing outpatient facilities at the beginning of the project and for years afterward.

Each physician invested $44,000 and became a general partner, thus requiring major decisions be made by majority vote. Each partner has equal liability for partnership debts. We elected a board of directors and hired a consultant to study the demographics of the area, project the caseload, and choose a site.

We selected a law firm to start the ball rolling. It seems fair to say that we could have done a better job of managing this extremely important decision. It seemed as if we would bear some risk no matter whom we selected because no other local law firm had experience developing such an entity. Indeed, there were probably few qualified firms in the entire nation at that time. Today there are many law firms with experience in this field, and there is no substitute for experience. But, at that time, we hired a lawyer who was a friend of one of the partners and who had done legal work for him. As time passed, some physician partners concluded that the lawyer was more interested in generating billable hours than in giving us good value for his services. We hired another lawyer.

We had to raise enough money from the partners to obtain bank loans and sustain the project during the inevitable cost overruns. Collecting sufficient funds from partners in the beginning also reduces the likelihood of having to make subsequent assessments. As the project progressed, it became necessary on several occasions to collect additional sums from the partners. The initial investment was $7,700 for developing the business, $16,500 for a separate real estate partnership, and a total of $19,800 in subsequent business assessments. Everyone complied, but imposing the assessments was a most unpleasant chore. The partnership saved some money by securing loans directly from banks without the services of a broker. Physicians contemplating this type of partnership should keep in mind that it is difficult to mobilize 30 partners to turn in their personal financial statements when the bank calls for them.

Escondido is a rapidly-growing inland area in north San Diego County. Tax-supported Palomar is the only hospital in the vicinity, and it serves a district with a population of 324,000. As we deliberated on our organizational structure, some physician partners urged us not to get involved with the hospital. Others wanted the hospital to participate to neutralize the administration's opposition to competition, and a partnership interest would allow the hospital to recoup some of the money it would lose on outpatient surgery. We eventually accepted that argument, but then the hospital itself decided not to join us. The hospital's attorney concluded that laws governing tax-supported hospitals precluded joint ventures with physicians. Of course, that legal opinion has shifted 180 degrees since those early days of physician entrepreneurial activity. Today Palomar is involved with several joint ventures with members of its medical staff.

But at that time, we achieved a compromise by contracting with Palomar to administer our facility, a move we expected would assure their support. With that arrangement, we could use hospital resources which the surgery center lacked, including equipment, gas sterilization, pharmacy services, and financial services. This relationship also helped us nail down an essential patient transfer agreement for those who might need inpatient care.

We found land near the hospital with access from a main thoroughfare that would be convenient for patients and most of the physicians. Unfortunately, problems with the topography raised our construction costs. The terrain was steep enough to make it more complicated and thus more expensive to build a one-story building with adequate parking and setbacks for landscaping. The board interviewed design firms and chose an architect who had never before designed a medical facility. The architectural committee decided it wanted more than a "box," and it liked the architect's concept of a building that would not seem like a hospital to patients. But we paid a price for the designer's inexperience with medical facilities. We have had problems with faulty heating and cooling systems, inadequate storage, wasted space, etc. During the design and construction phase, the committee devoted a great deal of time to supervising the project with no immediate financial reward. They understood that the payback would come later, when revenue started to flow. In addition to regular board meetings, the committee's three members each spent two to five hours a week handling day-to-day interaction with the architect and the contractors.

The board interviewed and hired a local contracting firm that had an excellent reputation after comparing it with a large San Diego firm. We got quality construction at lower cost—$3 million. It is important to choose a local contractor with a good track record in health facility construction. Work began in January 1985, and we wound up with a beautiful building that works quite well and is admired and enjoyed by the patients. It is an attractively designed facility with four operating rooms and 20 full-time employees. But during the first winter, the place was so cold in the mornings that we had to set up electric space heaters all over the building. Eventually, the whole system might have to be replaced.

Today, we use three of the four operating rooms to handle about 225 surgeries a month, including tonsillectomy and adenoidectomy, hernia repair, breast biopsy, arthroscopy, laser surgery, cataract extraction with lens implant, and 150 endoscopies a month. We leased a radiology and ultrasound suite to the radiology group, whose outpatient business has now outgrown the facility. The radiologists have moved into larger quarters elsewhere, but they still retain some services that are supportive of surgery. It has not yet been determined how the center will use the remaining space in the radiology suite.

The original agreement between the partnership and Palomar Medical Center was for the hospital to manage the facility. The partnership selected the professional staff (RNs, etc.), but they were employees of the hospital district and participated in the district's employee benefit package. The partnership reimbursed the district for all employee-related expenses, and the hospital was responsible for running the business office and collecting accounts receivable in a timely manner. The hospital district was paid a percentage of gross revenues for this service.

Unfortunately, the hospital administrative personnel seemed to have no management direction or commitment to the surgery center's success. They certainly did not appreciate the differences between running a hospital and a free-standing facility. On the revenue side, they had an inappropriate fee structure and a lackadaisical collections department. On the expense side, they had poor cost control and personnel management. For example, operating room personnel would order anything a doctor requested and work unnecessary overtime. This can get out of hand.

It became apparent that our accounts receivable were growing large and old because the hospital district executive responsible for the center had other obligations that distracted him from adequately supervising key employees. Collections were not meeting expenses, and liabilities were not being retired as rapidly as we hoped. The board again had to assess the partners. Debt to the hospital district was growing because it was to be paid a percentage of gross revenues as opposed to a percentage of collections. After much negotiating, the contract between the partnership and the hospital district was terminated, and while we avoided litigation, costs to the partnership were substantial and probably delayed profitability for a year or two.

The board saw this situation long before recommending to the partners that the contract be terminated because the district administrators repeatedly assured us the problems were being corrected. The board probably was remiss in not terminating the contract sooner. In retrospect, it seems that payments for administrative services should be based on track record only. The better the performance, the better the compensation. Today, the center is tightly managed by an anesthesiologist who is both medical director and business manager. He has a master's degree in hospital administration, a good business sense, and because he has been with us since the beginning he has learned the mistakes that shouldn't be repeated. Our collection rate is now high and accounts are paid timely.

The medical community's initial skepticism about investing in the project extended to referrals as well. At first, many non-partner physicians expressed doubts about patient safety and quality of care and refused to refer to the surgery center. Some were quite candid about not wanting to refer patients to a facility that was enriching competitors who had partnership interests. But with time these doubts dissipated. The facility now enjoys the loyalty of many non-owner physicians who realize their patients receive better care at a lower cost and in a more timely manner at the center.

The Escondido Surgery Center has a fully organized medical staff under the direction of the board of directors and a full-time medical director. The credentials committee and quality assurance committee meet once a month, and committees on infection control, laser surgery, pathological tissue, and intraocular lens implantation meet as needed. To be eligible for medical staff membership, physicians must be active staff members at a fully accredited hospital in San Diego County and carry a minimum level of medical liability coverage.

The partnership decided to apply for a state license so we would be eligible to care for Medicaid and Medicare patients in addition to private pay patients. We felt this would make the facility more marketable should we desire to sell it later. Many free-standing surgery centers never apply for a state license as they have no interest in treating Medicaid patients. This added to our construction difficulties because California licensed medical facilities must submit architectural plans to appropriate state agencies, such as the fire marshal. This can become expensive, time-consuming, and frustrating. The center essentially makes no profit on Medicaid patients, but we continue to serve them as a convenience to referring physicians who, we hope, will also send private patients to the center.

Although our initial experiences with the hospital administration were disappointing, in 1989 the partners agreed to sell a half-interest in the surgery center to the hospital, which now has a new administrator. This time, however, the partners have retained the power to oversee employees furnished by the hospital district and to veto objectionable policies. The medical director/business manager who turned the center around after our first experience with the hospital remains in that position.

In 1990, we anticipated monthly profits of $500 per partner. The keys to our success were the determination of the partners to see it through and the selection of individuals to manage the project from design to construction to operation—the medical director, the nursing manager, and the office manager. When operations begin at any new surgery center, the medical director and nursing manager must work closely together with the constant goal of improving the quality of care and enhancing efficiency. The business manager's primary task must be to improve the rate and timeliness of collections, a job on which the success of the entire project depends.

Free-standing ambulatory surgery centers are now common throughout the nation, and joint venturing with local hospitals or national surgery center chains has become standard. The reasons for this are varied, but they include surgery centers' fear that hospitals will be able to sign exclusive contracts with third-party payers despite the fact that free-standing surgery centers can deliver superior care at lower cost.

Those who would want to create physician-owned surgery centers in their own communities must be mindful of the potential threat of state and federal regulation that could affect their plans. A few years ago, Congress encouraged entrepreneurial physician activity as a way of injecting competition into the medical marketplace. I believe that many of these ventures have become successful financially because they filled a gap in the medical marketplace and offered a service the public wants and needs. Some physician-owned entities are alleged to be involved in unscrupulous or unethical business practices. I believe these to be a small minority. But because of this small minority, officials have proposed legislation to ban physician referrals to facilities in which they hold an ownership interest. Study the current laws and proposals in the legislative pipeline.

––––––––––––––––––

ALEX FRASER, M.D., received his undergraduate education at Iowa State University, Ames, and completed his medical education at University of Iowa College of Medicine (1967). After an internship at Sacramento County Hospital, California, Dr. Fraser completed his residency in anesthesiology at University of Virginia, Charlottesville. He followed this with a fellowship in anesthesiology at University of California, Davis, and then spent two years on active duty with the U.S. Navy Medical Corps. For the past 17 years he has been in the private practice of anesthesia at the Palomar Medical Center, Escondido, California. He is a Diplomate of the American Board of Anesthesiology and is a member of the California Society of Anesthesiologists, the American Society of Anesthesiologists, and the American Society of Regional Anesthesia. Dr. Fraser is a partner in the Escondido Surgery Center and is a member of the board of directors of the Cooperative of American Physicians, an inter-indemnity professional liability trust.

5

Saga of a Surgicenter

Alan E. Bickel, M.D.

The outpatient surgery center concept began in 1969 as the brainchild of two Phoenix anesthesiologists, Wallace Reed and John Ford, but it did not become generally accepted by the medical establishment for another decade. Before their innovation, almost 100 percent of surgery was performed on an inpatient basis, with patients admitted to hospitals the night before surgery and discharged no sooner than the day after the operation. These pioneers braved the hierarchy of the hospitals and accepted the challenge of justifying their beliefs to government agencies in order to gain permission to build and operate their facility.

Selling the concept to surgeons who were used to caring for patients only within the secure walls of the traditional hospital was an additional challenge, but within a year Drs. Ford and Reed were running a rousingly successful venture. Patient approval was almost instantaneous because of the typical patient sentiments: "You don't go to the hospital unless you're sick," and "I don't like hospitals." Patients found it far more palatable to have surgery away from a hospital setting—without sacrificing the medical safety of a hospital—and to complete their recovery at home. And because the same procedures in the outpatient setting usually cost 30 to 40 percent less than when performed in a hospital, the concept was easier to sell to third-party payers.

I was first exposed to the Phoenix surgery center concept while attending a medical meeting in 1973. I already had spent 17 years traveling daily from one hospital to another to administer anesthesia. During that entire period, I had been on obstetrical and surgical call several nights a week. The prospect of practicing in one location with almost all healthy patients, without emergency day or night call, was very appealing. Several months later, I contacted the Phoenix physicians and expressed an interest in visiting their center.

They invited another anesthesiologist and me to come from San Jose for a visit so we could evaluate whether such a facility would be viable in our area. We were warmly welcomed by the staff and its owners and spent two days absorbing all we could. We were impressed with the efficiency of care, the broad spectrum of procedures they performed, and the satisfaction of the patients. We returned to San Jose and enthusiastically approached our hospital administrator with the concept. But his response was less than enthusiastic. He promised to "look into it" and assigned a finance department intern to perform a feasibility study. In spite of repeated inquiries about the progress of the study, it was nearly a year before we learned the administration had looked at the report and decided not to become involved in such a project. We were very disappointed—not only at their final decision, but that it had taken them so long to reach it. But my colleague and I decided to press on.

At about that time, the founders of the Phoenix surgicenter called to tell us they hoped to work with anesthesiologists around the country setting up free-standing surgery centers on a franchise basis. Our loosely organized anesthesiology group in San Jose was built only around apportioning the call schedule and not business development. So two of us decided to proceed alone to create a San Jose surgery center in cooperation with the Phoenix group. During the following months we purchased an option on a site, commissioned building plans, filed papers of incorporation, and applied for a state certificate of need. But while awaiting the certificate of need, we learned that our two partners from Phoenix had severed their own business relationship and their dissolution was entangled in legal delays. Before they finished, our certificate of need expired. The San Jose corporation and our proposal died with it.

Within six months a new group was formed by one of the Phoenix physicians and I was contacted again. This group planned to build and operate outpatient surgery centers on a franchise basis working with local anesthesiologists as director-managers. Again months flew by as we investigated all aspects of the business venture. Although the hospital administrators had rejected us in the past, I believed we could gain more by working with them. So I again approached the hospital with an offer to lease a site on its campus, build and operate a facility using its nursing staff, and, donate it to the hospital after 20 years. Again the administrators were not interested, although by this time they had decided to create a two-operating room outpatient department in the hospital.

Although the chance to work with a franchise organization had advantages, such as its minimal financial commitment and a developed business plan, we decided we would be better off working independently. I decided to try to vitalize the hospital's new but lethargic outpatient unit by limiting my anesthesia practice solely to outpatient surgery. In one year outpatient volume increased more than 200 percent, with most cases receiving general anesthesia. This remarkable growth came about because surgeons and nursing staff saw that someone was committed to building and improving this service. It required only my commitment, not any particular talent or skills.

Two years later, the hospital became interested in building a free-standing outpatient center. It formed a committee and employed an attorney to secure a certificate of need. But after one year of legal and administrative action, the lawyer confided that the chances of approval appeared dismal. The hospital then experienced another revelation—they realized that physician-owned surgical centers did not require a certificate of need in California and several other states. They approached me with a familiar idea: organizing, building, and operating such a facility until they could purchase it. Working with a developer who had built large medical office complexes near the hospital, we pursued this approach and worked harmoniously with the hospital for several months.

But just as we reached the final stages of negotiation, the hospital declared its intent to purchase the building, land, and business on its own terms and at its own convenience. The developer and I had heard that song before, and we abruptly canceled all the plans. When this news reached the medical community I was approached by a fellow anesthesiologist who was building another surgical center across town. He offered me the opportunity to join him, but because of differing views on how to structure the business entity, I declined the offer. His proposal would have offered ownership only to anesthesiologists, and I believed that it was important to include surgeons to assure success.

About six months later, several other physicians and their business manager asked me to consider developing a surgical center in a medical office building a few blocks from two hospitals. The city had already approved a proposed two-story, 26,000-square-foot medical condominium on the site, and the first floor of the U-shaped building could probably house the surgical center. After more meetings with the group and an attorney, we formed a general-limited partnership and began to move rapidly with our plans. With only a moderate financial commitment from each physician, we prepared to develop a 10,700-square-foot space into the Los Gatos Surgery Center.

The space planner and architect consulted with us and designed a floor plan that allowed patients to enter at one end of the U and proceed smoothly and functionally through the pre-op area, surgery, and recovery room to discharge. The design preserved space for equipment storage, sterile supply, and clean and dirty workrooms. The remaining wing of the U became the staff lounge and dining room, which was separated from work areas and the recovery room.

Our next two decisions were perhaps the most important of all. We knew we personally didn't have the knowledge and skills necessary to package and operate the facility, so we set out to find and hire an experienced administrator who had been successful elsewhere. Through the grapevine we found a talented and knowledgeable nurse administrator who had helped launch a surgicenter in a nearby city and build it into a successful operation. We heard also that she might be available. Fortunately, she agreed to come aboard as a member of our staff and help guide us through our perilous beginning.

Our second important decision was not to limit ownership to the general partners (two obstetrician-gynecologists and two anesthesiologists) and to bring in 70 physicians from all surgical specialties as limited partners—the first such partnership of its size to develop an outpatient surgery center. Armed with our prospectus and business and building plans, we contacted reputable surgeons who had shown an interest in the outpatient surgery concept. In about four months we had 72 partners and the initial capitalization needed to secure a line of credit for operating capital, equipment loans from a local bank, and a construction loan from a savings and loan association. The partnership purchased the entire first floor. In retrospect, we should also have purchased the second floor for medical offices and kept sufficient space to add a recovery care facility, but at that time such a concept had not yet developed (see Chapter 11).

The director of nursing and I, as medical director, began formulating policies and procedures, ordering equipment and supplies, and interviewing and hiring employees. Fortunately our temporary quarters were nearby and we could easily monitor construction and modify the design as needed. The general partners met daily to make legal and building decisions. One key decision was to meet with a small group of gastroenterologists who asked us to consider an endoscopy room. In a vivid demonstration of what it means to be unfettered by bureaucracy, we were able within 30 minutes to design an endoscopy room to their specifications, something they had not been able to achieve at the hospital in more than three years. They were overjoyed, and so were we. Their utilization has been excellent since the surgery center became operational.

We planned to start employing the nursing staff a few weeks before opening, taking into consideration the usual construction delays. Before we held an open house, our nursing director, scheduling secretary, and office staff hosted a series of luncheons for nearby medical office staffs to meet them and acquaint them with the facility and its services. By the time we performed the first surgical procedure, more than 100 physicians had become credentialed members of our medical staff.

Although our facility houses four operating rooms equipped identically to those in a hospital, our initial caseload required only two rooms. We soon learned that most patients and surgeons desired their outpatient surgery on Thursdays and Fridays, thus allowing patients to recover over the weekend with minimal lost work time.

We were gratified when it took less than six months after starting operations to pass the break-even point, even though our fees were about 30 percent lower than the hospital. By our first anniversary we began to repay principal and reduce our debt.

Before opening, we applied for Medicare certification and were granted that status in the third month. Until the certification was actually issued, however, we were not paid by Medicare and Blue Cross for procedures performed on Medicare and Blue Cross patients. This was an expensive lesson for us and we have since passed it on to other developing facilities.

Physician and patient satisfaction with the center has been excellent. More than 95 percent of the patients who complete their evaluation cards describe the facility and the care in glowing terms. When negative responses and criticisms come in, we direct them to the involved department and consider how we might correct the problem. Employee satisfaction has been extremely high, with more than 90 percent of our original nursing and office personnel still working for the center after five years.

Always looking for opportunities to increase utilization and broaden our patient base, we considered a joint venture with a major neighboring hospital. After several months of meetings, the hospital requested that we meet with their consultant, "an expert in determining the value" of similar facilities. He presented his bid, but the offer could not be seriously considered. Almost a year later, we sold an interest in the center to a large health maintenance organization while retaining management and operating control. The neighboring hospital and a competing surgery center were not especially thrilled about the deal. However, we still cooperate and share equipment and supplies when necessary.

By our fifth anniversary, our medical staff had performed more than 22,000 procedures at the center. At the start of our venture, we were in the vanguard of the outpatient surgical movement. We believe we were among the first to form such a large partnership for a surgical center. Our partners take pride in offering their facility as an economical and high-quality alternative to hospital care. The medical staff participates in the delivery and planning of care without getting bogged down in endless committee work and unnecessary delays.

We continue to focus on improving our work attitudes, ethics, and patient services. Our goal is to create a customer-oriented atmosphere that shows through from the first telephone contact, through the patient's discharge, and afterward with the business office. We want our clients to say, "Those people really care about me!" Our patient-response cards, anonymous physician questionnaires, and internal critiques help us in this quality-assurance appraisal.

When we began our center, we benefited from the fact that California did not have a certificate of need requirement for physician-owned entities like ours. However, this did create several problems. We had no construction or facility operation guidelines from the state. Today surgical centers must be licensed and follow certain guidelines in planning their facilities.

Can others create similarly successful outpatient surgical center? The answer is, in fact, a resounding "Yes!" if they are willing to accept the financial risk, invest the time to assemble a core group of hard-working and knowledgeable medical, legal, administrative, and nursing professionals, and establish realistic goals. With the constant changes in health care delivery and third-party compensation, it is essential for physicians to remain adaptable and innovative in order to provide the best possible patient care at the lowest cost. It already is apparent that only the seriously ill patient and those requiring major surgery will continue to need the traditional hospital setting. Everyone else will be cared for in short-term, outpatient facilities. Physicians must invent solutions to the challenges spawned by this trend. We must not merely follow others in the march toward innovation, we must lead it!

ALAN E. BICKEL, M.D., received his undergraduate and medical school education from Northwestern University (M.D. 1953) in Evanston, Illinois. Following an internship at Blodgett Memorial Hospital, Grand Rapids, Michigan, he completed his residency in anesthesiology at Santa Clara County Hospital, San Jose, California. He has been in private practice in San Jose and Los Gatos since 1956. He was chairman of the department of anesthesia at Good Samaritan Hospital, San Jose, and currently is a general partner and medical director of the Los Gatos Surgical Center. He is a member of the American Society of Anesthesiology, the California Society of Anesthesiology, and the American Professional Practice Association. He is a founding director of the National Intercity Bank (Silicon Valley Bank) of Santa Clara, and a founding general partner of the Almaden Valley Athletic Club.

6

The BreastCare Center

By David Kramer, M.D.

Breast cancer has a mortality rate second only to lung cancer in women, and it has remained essentially unchanged for 60 years. About 140,000 new cases of invasive breast cancer are diagnosed annually, and about one in 10 women will develop the disease at some point during their lives. At least 35 percent of the women with invasive tumors die of the disease—about 40,000 Americans this year. Death rates for women over 50 have increased slightly over the past decade, and while no proven technologies have yet decreased the incidence of breast cancer, earlier detection has been shown to lower the associated mortality and morbidity. Screening mammography is currently the premier method of early detection of breast cancer.

The landmark studies that documented the efficacy of mammography screening are the Health Insurance Plan of Greater New York Screening Project and the Breast Cancer Detection Demonstration Project. Additional studies from Sweden and Holland have confirmed their conclusions.

The next step is to convince the public and members of the medical profession of the benefits of screening mammograms. The American Cancer Society has taken a strong leadership role in this educational campaign. By using press conferences, broadcast public service announcements, and press releases, the Cancer Society has targeted women—especially the elderly and minorities—for education about the importance of mammography and breast health guidelines. Also, by encouraging physicians to refer appropriately for screening, the Cancer Society hopes to bring more women into this early detection campaign.

A major part of the educational program directed to physicians is to promote the guidelines for mammography. The American Cancer Society recommends that all women have a baseline mammogram between the ages of 35 and 40 years. Women between 40 and 49 are urged to have annual or biennial screening mammograms. This should be done annually after 50 years of age. Women between the ages of 20 and 40 are advised to have a physical examination of the breast by a physician every three years, and annually when 40 or older. In addition, all women over 20 years old should be instructed and encouraged to conduct regular breast self-examination.

These guidelines have been endorsed by 10 prominent health care organizations, including the National Cancer Institute, the American Medical Association, the National Medical Association, the American College of Radiology, the American Society of Internal Medicine, the American Academy of Family Physicians, and the American Society for Therapeutic Radiology and Oncology.

Despite the publicity of these guidelines, physician acceptance of the value of screening mammography is seen as needing improvement. Only a small percentage of eligible women undergo mammography screening, with obstetricians and gynecologists more committed to screening than internists and family practitioners. "Too many physicians are withholding mammography in the absence of symptoms, at a time when the main purpose of mammography is to find the asymptomatic cancer," the American Cancer Society has stated. The greatest deterrents to screening mammography are the absence of physician recommendations and the patient's rejection of referral. A patient's compliance is directly affected by the presence of self-reported breast symptoms, abnormal findings on physical examination, and the source of payment for the test.

In 1986 and 1987, the American Cancer Society, together with groups of radiologists and the media, sponsored low-cost mammography screening projects in various locations throughout

Southern California. This campaign provided $50 mammograms to asymptomatic women over the age of 35. To qualify for the low-cost screening, a woman must have had no previous mammogram, no previous breast surgery or radiation therapy, no silicone injections or implants, and have exhibited no dominant breast lump or discharge. She also could not be pregnant or lactating, and must have been referred by a physician to whom the results could be sent. More than 20,000 mammograms were performed under this ACS program.

Surveys conducted at other screening mammography sites have shown that a unique opportunity exists at a project site for data collection and dissemination of educational information. These surveys have shown no consistent relationship between a woman's age and her use of the service, although they noted a higher utilization rate by better educated women. Although there is no difference in use between Caucasians and blacks, other races are considerably less likely to undergo screening mammography. Women in metropolitan areas use mammography more regularly than those in the suburban or rural areas. Jewish women have a much higher usage rate than any other religious group. Women with annual incomes exceeding $15,000 are more likely to undergo mammography than those with lower incomes. Involvement in other health activities, including breast self-examination, is also associated with increased usage, as is prior knowledge of breast cancer detection, treatment options, and mortality rates.

As anticipated, the American Cancer Society's low-cost screening projects have generated considerable public interest in routine mammograms. Physicians in the San Jose, California, area reported a fivefold increase in patient requests for mammograms and an increased appetite for breast cancer information. In order to meet these demands, the San Jose Medical Center instituted a feasibility study for developing a breast care center where low-cost screening mammograms and patient education services would be offered. By dedicating a space to this specialized area of health care, the medical center believed that this service could be provided efficiently and with high quality. Because San Jose is also a highly competitive medical community, the medical center saw an added advantage in developing a screening facility—increased public awareness of the medical center.

As part of this feasibility study, the medical center conducted two focus groups on women's health concerns. Topics included attitudes about women's medical care, provider preferences, and the prospect of a women's center. In the focus groups, most women expressed concern about their health and their desire to be better educated about potential health problems. The study also suggested that women prefer to use an aesthetically pleasing, free-standing women's center for their care.

Based on this mini-market survey, the medical center organized a task force with the medical staff to discuss a joint-venture breast care center. This task force included representatives from the hospital-based radiology partnership, the South Bay Medical Group (an independent practice association with 220 physicians), and the San Jose Medical Group (a 60-member multispeciality clinic). The inclusion of all components of the medical staff on the task force was seen as essential.

The agenda for the task force was an open discussion of the proposed breast care center's services, including self-referral arrangements, reimbursement, screening guidelines, facility ownership, location, and whether the unit should be mobile or fixed. No other comprehensive program of breast cancer screening then existed near the medical center, so a survey of patients who had used San Jose Medical Center in the past was conducted to determine their reaction to such a breast center. Routine diagnostic mammography services were being offered at two nearby locations and were priced at the usual rate, which was considerably higher then the fee proposed for the screening mammography at the breast care center. This survey helped the task force identify the strengths and weaknesses of existing mammography services and tailor a proposal that would account for the effects of competition.

The task force decided to develop the San Jose BreastCare Center within the hospital's radiology department, and to offer screening mammograms for $75, about 60 percent of the usual fee in the community. A limited partnership was created with the San Jose Medical Center as the general partner. On May 18,

1988, an offer to participate in the limited partnership was mailed to members of the medical staff. The offering was for 50 limited partnership units priced at $2,900 each. The partnership hired a national health care consulting firm to organize the offering and to provide administrative and accounting services.

The BreastCare Center was initially capitalized with $146,465, of which 99 percent came from the limited partners. Expenses were $75,950 for medical equipment; $30,000 for organizational costs; $30,000 for brokerage fees; and $10,515 for capital reserves. The partnership purchased a Senographe 500T dedicated mammography system manufactured by Thomson-CGR Medical Corporation, a subsidiary of General Electric Company. A second unit is scheduled to be acquired in 1990.

State-of-the-art equipment is essential, and reproducibly optimum mammograms made within an acceptable radiation dose are mandatory. With mass screening, the screen film system is more efficient and less expensive per image than with xeromammography because of the capacity for faster processing. This equipment required a molybdenum target x-ray tube with a 0.3-mm to 0.6-mm focal spot, which prolongs tube life. A smaller focal spot is not required because magnification views are not necessary in the screening setting.

The partnership purchased the equipment and leased it to the medical center for the screening mammography services. The partnership is paid a fixed fee by the medical center for each mammogram conducted. The fees to the medical center are cost-accounted so the hospital can perform the mammograms at a competitive price. The medical center is the actual provider of services for billing and licensing purposes, and it is responsible for the day-to-day operations. As the general partner, the medical center is accountable to the limited partners for profits and losses, and it assumes financial liability if the partnership fails.

The medical center established the BreastCare Center in a remodeled portion of the radiology department and assigned a technical staff to operate it. The BreastCare Center, therefore, has a distinct identity. Mammogram interpretation is performed by the medical center's radiology group within 24 hours. Most patients (97 percent) are referred to the center by their physician, with only 3 percent of the patients self-referred. Women who have no physician are referred after the examination to members of a physician panel. If a malignancy is suspected or suggested by the mammograms, the center sends the patient a registered letter urging her to seek medical follow-up.

With a charge of $75, including the professional component, the BreastCare Center immediately became the price leader in Santa Clara County, and other mammography practices have lowered their prices to remain competitive. This was unexpected, but from the public's perspective, it was a welcome benefit.

The medical center adopted a promotional plan that built awareness and usage of its program among women's groups in the San Jose metropolitan area. The center distributed 20,000 brochures, aired public service radio spots, and conducted press conferences. The new program was announced to management, employees, and the medical staff. An open house was held for medical staff members and administration. On-site luncheons were held for physician office staffs, business women, and women's clubs. The program was marketed to athletic clubs and at health fairs. The BreastCare Center is promoted in the newspaper regularly.

Special attention was given to medical staff members. After the appropriate specialties were identified, each physician received brochures and ordering pads along with an explanation of the program. The explanation contained details of the examination, its indications, follow-up methods, and a list of known risk factors for breast cancer. Each physician received a personal letter from a radiologist involved in the interpretation of the mammograms. After the program was open, the center solicited feedback, and it regularly communicates any changes in the program with physicians. Presentations were made to each of the appropriate medical staff departmental meetings.

During the first 16 months of operation, an average of 110 mammograms were performed each month. Although this average of five examinations per day is lower than original projections, the limited partners have had a small return on their investment and are especially pleased with the quality of the program and responses from their patients. About 30 percent of the referrals to the San Jose BreastCare Center are from the offices of limited partners.

The BreastCare Center considers education of the physician to be an important goal if screening mammography is to have its fullest impact in the early detection of breast cancer. To help increase physician awareness of the screening test, the unit's staff was carefully instructed in responding to the major concerns of the medical staff. These concerns include:

Risk of radiation. The American Cancer Society has concluded that "modern technology has reduced the radiation exposure of low-dose mammography to the point of negligible risk, if risk exists at all, and has increased its diagnostic capabilities at the same time."

Unnecessary biopsies. The number of biopsies has increased, but they are more apt to find an early, non-invasive cancer that is highly curable. Only about one in five biopsies for a suspicious mammographic finding currently will show a cancer.

Over-diagnosis. Screening mammograms will often detect breast cancer at the pre-clinical stage, when it is not detected by palpation, either by the patient or by the physician. Although some older patients may never become symptomatic, it must be assumed that most of these cancers eventually will cause morbidity and mortality.

Cost. In screening mammography facilities with a high volume of studies, costs can be kept low. Because greater detail is sometimes needed, there may be additional films and other costs for suspicious findings. The cost-benefit ratio must be viewed from the perspective of reducing overall morbidity and mortality. The vast majority of women do not require additional views.

Scheduling the examination as soon as is convenient for the patient is a high priority, and it can usually be performed within 24 hours of the request from the physician's office. When the woman is scheduled for the screening examination, her menstrual cycle is considered to minimize any discomfort with the exam. Women are advised to avoid caffeine for 24 hours prior to the study. At the time of the examination, a technologist conducts a breast health history in a private and comfortable surrounding. Any questions are answered, and educational material is made available. Each patient then views a short videotape demonstrating the technique of proper breast self-examination. If desired by the patient, she can work with models simulating breast tissue and breast lumps.

The mammography room need not be large, but it should be comfortable and decorated pleasantly. Two screening projections of each breast are made, and if any abnormality is detected, the patient should be referred for a more comprehensive study. Using well trained technical staff and photo-timed exposures reduces the technical problems that necessitate a recall of the patient for re-screening.

"Batch processing" of the films at the end of the day facilitates faster service to patients. The mammograms are read by board-certified radiologists at the end of the day or the next morning, and a report is available to the patient's physician within 24 hours.

The center requests that payment be made at the time of the examination, a policy that significantly reduces billing and accounting costs.

The anticipated benefits of the BreastCare Center extend well beyond the financial returns to the partners. The medical center expects it to increase new referrals for related hospital services, the net results of which may far outweigh the revenue from the screening program itself. Original volume projections were based on results of similar programs, advice of the consultants, and the cumulative effect on the population to be served and the ownership interest of the physician limited partners. The limited partners' priority goal for the BreastCare Center is to provide high-quality screening services at an affordable cost to patients.

The medical center has been very receptive to the limited partners' suggestions about improving various aspects of the BreastCare Center. The partners are determined to maintain a high quality of care and to keep patients satisfied with the study and the ambience of the facility itself. The program is seen as being of relatively low risk for the medical center because of its low capital investment. The "bonding effect" created by this joint venture is considered very worthwhile by the medical center.

The BreastCare Center at the San Jose Medical Center has received wide physician and patient acceptance. The publicity, especially in the newspapers, has made women more aware of screening mammography as the superior method for early detection of breast cancer. The low cost of the study has drawn many women to the center for their baseline mammograms, something they had been postponing because of the cost. During the examination, women are provided with excellent information, reinforcing the need for early detection and regular self-examination. The BreastCare Center has enhanced the medical center's reputation in the community as being concerned with the health and well being of the people in San Jose and throughout the surrounding South Bay area.

DAVID KRAMER, M.D., received his undergraduate education (A.B., 1964) at Hunter College, Bronx, New York, and his medical education at the State University of New York at Buffalo School of Medicine. He completed his internship and residency in radiology at Rochester General Hospital, Rochester, New York, following which he was on the faculty of the University of Michigan Hospital as a radiology instructor. He served two years in the U.S. Air Force stationed at McClellan Air Force Base, Sacramento, California. Since 1976, he has been in the private practice of radiology in San Jose, California. Dr. Kramer is a diplomate of the American Board of Radiology and is active in the California Radiological Society, the American College of Radiology, and the Radiological Society of North America. He is on the editorial board of the CE/Q Medical Newsletter.

7

Acute Health Care at Home

Mary Griffin, R.N., M.P.H.

The unprecedented growth of managed health care and prospective payment systems in the early 1980s revolutionized
American health care. For the first time, the nation had an excellent reason to consider alternatives to the longterm hospitalization of Medicare patients. But even before Medicare adopted
prospective payments in 1983, many third-party payers knew
that relentless and steep hospital cost inflation would force the
nation to find alternatives that would keep the system from hur-
tling out of control.

In 1985, I joined a group of investors and managers who recognized an opportunity to reinvent a service that had been around
for a long time but always had been taken for granted. Home
health care for many years had been used primarily as an adjunct
to hospitalization instead of as a genuine alternative to it. Our
group knew we could devise ways to treat high-acuity patients
at about half the cost of hospitalization in an environment that
was more comfortable, convenient and sanitary, and that was
based on a wellness model instead of a sickness model. We knew
we could move patients to their own homes under the care of
licensed professional nurses and under the direction of their physicians. This was a new concept, and at times it would require
a rather radical approach. Our goals were to:

• Bring patients with very high acuity needs into their homes
sooner than usual.

- Continue to provide them with high-quality, cost-effective care.
- Involve physicians in our company.
- Ask physicians and third-party payers to delineate which services they wanted and needed and tell us how we could simplify their jobs.

The traditional home care model evolved from public health nursing of the late nineteenth century. Nurses then served homebound invalids, the elderly, and patients with chronic and communicable diseases in a model that virtually excluded active physician participation. When Congress passed the Medicare laws in 1965 and extended coverage to home health care, the U.S. Health Care Financing Administration created a package of benefits modeled on the antiquated public health "visiting nurse." This became the standard of practice for hundreds of government, non-profit, and proprietary home health agencies nationwide, but it is now obsolete.

Because Medicare was the No. 1 buyer of home health services, various trade organizations focused their lobbying efforts on supporting the visiting nurse model—to the detriment of home health providers whose services fell outside the narrow coverage definitions set down by Medicare. Some companies provided attendants or nurses' aides to the elderly, but because Medicare didn't cover those services, it made no attempt to regulate the care. Thus many developed reputations for rendering poor care and overcharging or abusing the elderly. Other agencies provided "private duty" licensed nurses to care for patients at home, but many of these nurses were recruited out of retirement or from skilled nursing facilities, and they were not as current and sophisticated as nurses working in acute-care hospitals. As a result, private duty agencies often were criticized for providing inadequate care and failing to communicate with the physician. Both types of companies had recognized that some patients' needs couldn't be met by the visiting nurse model, but Medicare's only answer to them was hospitalization.

In March 1985, our group, the Home Hospital Corporation, developed a division called HomeMed of America Incorporated to provide high-quality home services in a way that would satisfy patients, physicians, and payers. Our diverse board of directors included a real estate developer who wanted to build alternative living facilities for the elderly; a certified public accountant who wanted to create a company to deliver high-acuity alternative care to children at home; an attorney who had been vice-president of a national home care company; and a surgeon who had used traditional home health care services for post-operative patients.

We began by asking some basic questions: Why are patients being kept in the hospital after they are stabilized if their primary need is good nursing supervision and care? What types of patients can be managed at home? How much would it cost to provide all the services needed to maintain a patient at home? Would third-party payers recognize the savings of home care and offer it as a benefit? Would physicians be willing to discharge patients with high-acuity needs directly from the hospital to home care? How would patients and families respond to home care as an alternative to hospitalization? How difficult would it be to recruit qualified nurses? How would the hospitals react, and what effect would it have on their relationship with physicians? How could we identify patients early in their hospital stays who are suitable for high-acuity home care?

Our first step was to find physicians who would be interested in proving our theories. We chose a 150-physician group practicing in a prestigious medical clinic in Northern California. Physicians from virtually every specialty work in the clinic and serve a population mixed in age and payment sources.

Then the real work began. We put on our most comfortable shoes and our thickest skins and began educating physicians in the best use of a new kind of home care company. Most were receptive to the traditional public health home care model but uncomfortable about substituting high-acuity home services for hospitalization. We sought their active participation by encouraging them to ask questions and express concerns—and did we hear concerns! "How will I know how my patient is doing unless I go to the home, too?" "What if there is an emergency in the home? How will it be handled, and by whom?" "Can I be sued for sending my patient home when other patients with the same condition are staying longer in the hospital?" "Can I trust the home-care nurses?" "What revenues will I lose by not being able to visit patients in the hospital?" "Will I get after-hour calls at home about my patients?"

To answer those questions, we developed case summaries to demonstrate the conditions we had handled in the home. The physicians could relate to the examples and focus on the specific clinical implications instead of hypothetical situations. The case studies also helped us define specific issues and take them up separately. Here are three examples:

Diagnosis: Cancer of the colon.

Home care needs: Nursing services, supplies and equipment, IV fluids, lab.

Case progress: A 60-year-old female had a loop colostomy performed for a bowel obstruction secondary to colon cancer. She was discharged home with one-to-one nursing care for fluid replacement, control of nausea and pain, assessment of gastro-intestinal functioning, care of Salem sump tube to suction, and ostomy care. Care was decreased as the family became knowledgeable about symptom management and colostomy care.

Actual length of hospitalization:	3.0 days	$1,800
Alternative acute care:	3.0 days	1,620
Total hospital and alternative care:	6.0 days	3,420
Previous average hospital stay:	8.3 days	4,980
Net savings:	2.3 days	1,560

Comments: Alternative care can be used to avoid unnecessary rehospitalization of patients suffering from pain, nausea, and fluid imbalance commonly associated with oncology. Alternative acute care also can provide IV chemotherapy in the home to avoid institutionalization.

Diagnosis: Spinal cord injury; quadriplegia.

Home care needs: Nursing, therapy, supplies and equipment, pharmacy, lab.

Case progress: A 23-year-old female with quadriplegia following a traumatic spinal cord injury required home ventilator care upon discharge from the hospital. Prior to discharge, the RN case manager and the respiratory therapist assessed the home environment and set up a plan and equipment for discharge. The nursing staff, which initially provided 24-hour care, was introduced to the patient and family and trained in the operation of the equipment and the patient's routine. Once home, the patient was prepared for routine oximetry and radiology tests, and the family was instructed in care needs. As the patient and family became competent in providing ongoing care, the nurses were discontinued and attendant care was substituted.

Actual length of hospitalization:	14 days	$10,500
Alternative acute care stay:	10 days	5,400
Total hospital and alternative care:	24 days	15,900
Previous average hospital stay:	28 days	21,000
Net savings:	4 days	5,100

Comments: A wide variety of injuries can be handled with alternative acute care far more cost effectively than in a hospital. Where appropriate, alternative acute care can provide home care while the patient awaits admission to a rehabilitation program.

Diagnosis: Prematurity, bronchopulmonary dysplasia.

Home care needs: Nursing services, IV antibiotics, supplies and equipment, oxygen, nebulizer, lab.

Case progress: A female born 12 weeks premature with respiratory distress syndrome required mechanical ventilation. She was discharged home with 24-hour nursing care. She required oxygen at 1 liter per minute per cannula, gavage feedings, multiple medications, and close assessment for respiratory distress.

At home, the parents learned to assume care of the infant, and services were downgraded to respite care only. All necessary equipment and the pediatric physical therapist for developmental therapy was arranged through alternative acute care.

Actual length of hospitalization:	25 days	$30,000
Alternative acute care stay:	20 days	16,800
Total hospital and alternative care:	45 days	46,800
Previous average hospital stay:	58 days	69,600
Net savings	13 days	22,800

Comments: Use of alternative acute care services opened up a neonatal intensive care unit bed for other newborns and helped bring this infant to its home environment sooner.

Most patients remain in the hospital because they need good nursing care and because physicians require accurate and timely feedback on patient status. We can fulfill both needs with the patient at home at about half the cost and with higher quality. The nurse provides one-to-one nursing care, observes changes in patient status immediately, and reports them to the physician. Most emergencies can be dealt with quickly and efficiently by the nurse alone.

The strongest factor influencing physicians' desire to use home care is neither personal financial interest in HomeMed nor philosophical support for the benefits of home care, but the physicians' own convenience. Do we make it convenient for them to refer patients to us? Can they obtain information about patient status whenever they need it? Early on we had to convince physicians that our nurses were easily accessible and that off-hours contacts would be minimal. If the physician finds it less convenient to use home care than to keep the patient in the hospital, the patient will probably stay in the hospital. Some physicians who use HomeMed earn fewer fees for hospital visits, but that gives them more time to devote to office visits and to admit other patients to the hospital.

After consulting with the physicians, we developed contingency emergency protocols and procedures specific to each patient. From experience, we know that once the patient is home and under the close supervision of highly qualified nurses, situations requiring after-hours calls to physicians rarely arise. When direct physician services are required, our nurses transport patients to the physicians' offices for examination and treatment. All lab workups are done at home, and results are reported immediately to the physician.

We believe that HomeMed's success depends on building a high-quality nursing staff that everyone can trust. They simply have to be the best. Most of our nurses have backgrounds in critical care. Many work part-time for our company and part-time for hospitals, so their clinical skills are current. HomeMed nurses have backgrounds in neonatology, pediatrics, oncology, medicine-surgery, orthopedics, rehabilitation, and most other specialties. We spend more on staff recruitment, training, and supervision than on any other item, and that separates us from other home care providers. We thoroughly interview each nurse and check all references. Some nurses working in hospitals do not pass our rigorous evaluation process. The RNs who do qualify attend orientation meetings, where they learn that they must participate in continual in-service training.

HomeMed opened for business in a 400-square-foot office in Palo Alto in September, 1985, with a nursing director, a staffing coordinator, and a secretary. Today, our company has 150 employees, including a full-time staff of about 40. We work out of offices in Menlo Park, Los Angeles, and Irvine, and with the help of contractors we cover 20 counties in California.

As soon as we started, it was apparent that the expertise of HomeMed's nurses matched or surpassed that of their hospital colleagues. HomeMed nurses have been trained to assess each patient thoroughly and to monitor and document all changes in patient status. They communicate with attending physicians by telephone and in writing as often as requested. Physicians have developed trust and respect for our nurses. When we began seeing handwritten notes from physicians complimenting our nursing staff, we knew our hiring and training policies were working.

HomeMed finds it relatively easy to hire qualified nurses because of the diversity of the work, the high degree of autonomy they enjoy on the job, and the variety of working situations available. Nurses can choose continuous care or move about from one type of patient to another. We have noticed that some hospital-based nurses have difficulty adjusting to home care because they lose some of their unchallenged authority. In the patient's home, the nurse is a guest, not an enforcer.

Third-party payers needed encouragement to give home health care a chance as a hospital alternative. Most home health agencies had focused almost exclusively on Medicare as the payer and ignored large insurers, workers compensation carriers, health maintenance organizations, and other managed care organizations. We set out to develop a service we could sell to all these payers. At the time, we knew of no other health care provider that had attempted to include physicians in management functions and approach payers with radical new concepts in patient care.

But as we made the rounds, we heard familiar questions and new concerns from the payers. "What if there is an emergency in the home?" "What kind of experience and training do HomeMed nurses have?" "Are physicians liable if something happens to the patient at home?" "Will the inclusion of a home-care benefit increase our costs?" "How do you stop home-care services once a patient and family grow accustomed to them?" "Will it cost more than keeping the patient in the hospital at our discounted per diem rates?" "How will we get the physician and patient to accept home care instead of hospitalization?"

Once again, we chose real-life examples from the payers' own experience or current files to identify appropriate home care candidates. We explained our emergency policies, hiring practices, and relationships with the physicians. We described how our services usually cost less than hospital per diems because we did not have to maintain a building, a dietary department, or a physical therapy unit. Our "team goals agreement," accepted by the payer, the patient, and the family, helps eliminate unrealistic patient and family expectations regarding the service period. The agreement lists the number of hours and days of service per week and the number of weeks included. This memorandum has practically eliminated patient anxiety and dependence on home care when patients are ready for discharge from our services.

Our organization trains the staff to teach patients and their families to provide self-care and move rapidly toward independence. This process begins before the patient leaves the hospital and is discussed at the discharge planning meeting and in the team goals agreement. This was a pivotal selling point for the payers because they realized that we were not planning to care for the patient indefinitely but were actively working toward an early and appropriate discharge from our care.

Physicians and payers now acknowledge that our services are unique and cost-effective—and certainly beneficial to patients. During our initial visit they always seem certain they have no patients who could use our services. We often ask if they had any patients currently in the hospital, in stable condition, who had a home to go to. When the answer is yes, we know we are dealing with a lack of physician understanding. We had to develop a system of identifying appropriate home-care candidates and participating in discharge planning.

Our management team uses nurses, who have experience and expertise in patient assessment, to help identify those patients who qualify for HomeMed service. This is our Proactive Case Management program and we offer it to physicians and payers. Our nurses go to the hospital to evaluate a patient referred by the physician or payer and prepare a patient care option report. In preparing this report, they apply an interdisciplinary approach involving the physician, other providers, the payer, the employer, risk management representatives, and the patient. The recommended options range widely, including leaving the patient in the hospital; discharging the patient to a skilled nursing facility or rehabilitation center; sending the patient home with home care services; or releasing the patient with no plans for follow-up services.

Our nurses do all of the discharge planning, service coordination, and follow-up care for patients referred to our program.

This program has become so successful that many payers request these services for patients out of our service area. We now perform Proactive Case Management for payers throughout California.

To help physicians and payers identify those patients appropriate for home care, we have established programs categorized by medical specialty. The following group of cornerstone programs is the foundation on which all our specialty programs are based:

Alternative Acute Care: Nurses provide round-the-clock, in-home care at the bedside in conjunction with therapies, pharmacy, equipment, lab, and x-ray to shorten hospital stays and speed recovery and patient independence.

Antibiotic Therapy: Skilled IV nurses instruct patient and family about antibiotic therapy, maintain IV sites, draw blood for lab studies, and remain available as needed to administer multiple doses. Clinical pharmacists provide the physician with a pharmacokinetics profile to ensure optimal drug therapy.

Home Hospital-Plus: Specialists provide on-site alternative care management, assess patient needs, write a care plan, and manage utilization.

Hospice Care: A medically directed, interdisciplinary team assesses patients with end-stage illnesses, provides support services, and counsels patients and families.

Nutritional Therapy: Highly skilled nursing staff provide comprehensive care, including nutritional assessment, patient and family education, and instruction about parenteral and enteral therapy. That training includes catheter or tube care, pump function, and administration, use, and storage of solutions. The 24-hour availability of nurses allows continuous monitoring. Lab studies and clinical pharmacy consultation ensure optimal therapy.

Pain Management: Specialized nurses educate patients and families about pain management and demonstrate administration of pain medications and maintenance of an IV site. Nurses achieve maximum pain control through close monitoring—round-the-clock if necessary.

Respite Care: Skilled nurses or attendants give families a break from caring for an ailing loved one.

Wound/Skin Care: Nurse specialists provide state-of-the-art wound care and infection control. Patients are educated in self-care and monitored until healing is complete.

Within these basic programs, the following specialty services are most often requested:

Oncology: AIDS management, chemotherapy infusion, family stress reduction, fluid replacement, Hickman catheter care, home transfusion, nausea control, self-stomal care, tube care.

Pulmonology: Arterial blood gas monitoring, asthma management, chest physiotherapy, environmental assessment, home respiratory care, oximetry monitoring, pulmonary rehabilitation, radiology-at-home, transtracheal oxygen.

Pediatrics-neonatology: BPD recovery, chemotherapy infusion, cystic fibrosis management, developmental assessment, fluid replacement, high-risk infant nutrition, home cardiorespiratory monitoring, home phototherapy, home traction, home ventilator, laboratory services, orthopedic rehabilitation, welcome-home infant assessment.

Surgery: Burn recovery, fluid replacement, home transfusion, wound care, laboratory services, mastectomy recovery, pre-operative education, pressure-sore recovery, post-operative nausea control, self-stomal care, short-stay surgery recovery, tube care.

We also devised specialty programs in orthopedics, gastroenterology, obstetrics-gynecology, infectious disease, internal medicine, and gerontology.

Many payers have complained to us about their experiences in trying to coordinate services to allow a patient to go home. They recount the confusion and time involved in calling a nursing service, a pharmacy, a medical supplier, a durable medical equipment firm, and a laboratory service. They talk about how difficult it is to work with so many providers and make sure the patient receives necessary services. They are troubled by the task of evaluating many providers and negotiating rates with each.

By offering all the necessary services through our local offices and quoting one price for the package, we resolve this problem. Our price includes nursing, infusion pharmacy, durable medical equipment, and laboratory and x-ray services. Physicians and payers need only make one call to our local office. The payer is charged a per diem rate based on the needs of the patient and the service required, and that rate is 30 to 40 percent lower than hospital rates.

Payers have begun to understand and use our services more frequently. They are particularly interested in oncology programs that keep patients with end-stage illnesses out of the hospital. Our neonatal programs allow infants with conditions of prematurity, such as bronchopulmonary dysplasia, cardiac defects, and congenital anomalies, to leave the neonatal intensive care unit sooner and move to the developmentally appropriate home environment. Early post-operative discharge programs allow patients to go home less than 48 hours after surgery. The short-stay surgery recovery program provides transportation home and nursing care for the first eight to 24 hours post-operatively. Physicians and payers requested our Welcome Home Post-Partum Program, which allows mothers and newborns to go home 12 hours after delivery. Our nurses follow up to assess them and instruct the mother in infant care.

We have created a complete, integrated system by listening to physicians and payers' requests for services and responding with programs that are easy to obtain. By our second year, we had developed strong working relationships with more than 400 physicians and signed contracts with most of the major payers in California. With so many different services in our repertoire and demand increasing, we needed a sophisticated management information system to track HomeMed divisions, partnerships and services. We wanted a system that could generate data that would be shared with payers to show the savings compared with hospital care. The system would need to be integrated with our operations and financial departments.

It took us a year to customize an integrated in-house computer system to monitor every patient referral from intake to discharge; every service provided; the revenues generated from each patient account; the cost of services; the physicians who referred the patients; the payers that referred the cases; and the profit earned on them. We linked our operation to the finance department and integrated accounts payable, accounts receivable, payroll, billing, and our financial statements. This system allows HomeMed to track every nurse and therapist who "touches" the patient and ascertain the number of hours spent on patient care, paperwork, travel, telephone calls, etc. We can calculate the cost of staffing each case and the number of hours of overtime, double time, holiday, vacation, and sick leave.

We can generate reports showing payers diagnosis related groups and ICD-9 codes for each patient and then compare the average length of stay and cost of hospitalization to the cost of home care. Our physician partners receive reports showing which patients they have on service, their diagnoses, the types of service their patients are receiving, the cost of the services, and the revenues generated by them.

This allows us to document home care cost savings, and, more importantly, to demonstrate how patients recuperate more rapidly at home. We were pleased to learn that patients often are discharged from our care ahead of schedule because they recover so much faster at home. For medical conditions that average five or six hospital days, we often take the patient home on Day Two and discharge by Day Three or Four with no other care needed. Not only has hospital time decreased by more than half, the total duration of care, including home health care, has dropped 40 to 50 percent.

The success of our Proactive Case Management Program has allowed us to expand through a statewide network of home care providers. We evaluate agencies for their ability to provide high-acuity services, and then HomeMed sets up protocols for the delivery of high quality care at home. The major challenge of building a network of contract providers is winning acceptance of the primary referral sources—especially payers, which account for 70 percent of HomeMed referrals. We remain involved in the supervision of care and assure clients that subproviders are as good as our own employees. In fact, HomeMed wields such a profound influence over the performance of contractors that we are tremendously confident about their work.

We are now able to service patients throughout California. In December, 1989, we opened our Sacramento office in a joint venture with Sutter Health Systems. This office provides alternative high-acuity home health services to Sutter's outpatients and acute care patients in Sacramento and surrounding areas. Our computer system and service technologies keep us on the cutting edge of alternative high-acuity services, and we are preparing to enter the national market. Our services have been refined to the point that we can enter other states and provide state-of-the-art care in a relatively short time.

HomeMed has been profitable every year since it began operating, achieving margins of up to 15 percent. The company had to make a conscious decision to control growth during 1989 to assure adequate controls over the rapidly expanding operation. Our division expects $5 million in gross revenue in 1989. This success is due to our willingness to listen. Clients, physicians, payers, and patients want us to offer one-stop shopping, provide case management and consultation, give per diem rates for services, and develop condition-specific programs. These programs have contributed to our leadership in alternative care delivery. We have vertically integrated services to cross-feed our business through our own programs. We continue to adapt and refine our services to meet client needs.

A working relationship requires trust, time, and effort. Selling your concepts and ideas is easy; getting people to use your services is not. We learned to accept the fact that no matter what you say or do and no matter how right you think it would be for them, some people will never want or use your service. We learned that hard work is not the only ingredient of success. Forbearance, persistence, patience, and the love of your task may be even more important.

We will continue to listen to our clients, for they have sparked our most innovative ideas. The health care world has changed dramatically during the last 20 years, and we expect it to change even more significantly in the next 20. The alternative care systems of today will be the traditional systems of tomorrow, and we look forward to developing new alternatives to meet the nation's changing needs.

———————————

MARY GRIFFIN, R.N., M.P.H., received her undergraduate education at San Jose State University (B.S., 1974), and completed graduate studies at Johns Hopkins University (M.P.H., 1983). After four years of hospital and public health nursing experience, she served as a nursing consultant for the Regional Center of the East Bay, Oakland, California. In 1983 she became the regional director for personal care health services in San Francisco. Since then, Ms. Griffin has been president of HomeMed of America Incorporated, Menlo Park, California, where she supervises the 150-employee Home Health Nursing Division of Home Hospital Corporation, an Alternative Healthcare Provider. She has lectured extensively to medical foundations, associations, and insurance companies on home health care as an alternative to acute in-hospital care. Ms. Griffin is available as a consultant in this unique field of health care.

8

The InfusiCenter Clinic

Paul F. Scholtes, M.S., M.S., J.D., and
Julia Sherman, B.S. (Pharm.)

InfusiCenter Clinics are outpatient facilities that enable physicians to convert two or three-day inpatient complex infusion treatments into one-day stays in a home-like environment. The concept grew out of Home Hospital Corporation's desire to better serve cancer patients and has been expanded to a wide range of other patient treatment applications. Physicians can send their patients for clinically excellent care in a warm, home-like environment instead of an institutional setting.

The concept incorporates the latest in clinical protocols and facility design. In contrast to the institutional feel of a hospital, the InfusiCenter Clinic looks like a bed and breakfast inn. It is large enough to include state-of-the-art technology, yet small enough to allow personal attention for patients and professional support for physicians because of the high staff-to-patient ratio. Located in physician office buildings, the clinics offer convenience to patients and families as well as to physicians who want to drop in on their patients during therapy.

The InfusiCenter Clinic's patient amenities are first-class and include tastefully decorated therapy suites with comfortable brass beds and plush comforters. The patient gazes upon oak moldings and floral wallpaper instead of stark white hospital walls. Soft lighting illuminates country oak furniture, flowers, and art work. Patients may watch television, read, or listen to a wide selection of music played on individual stereo systems during the typical

10- to 12-hour treatment day. The clinic is designed to be a low-volume, "high-touch" facility.

Cancer patients requiring extended chemotherapy infusions are generally not well-suited to home care because they need supervision and a safe, controlled environment. Yet the intensity of care for these patients usually does not warrant hospitalization. The InfusiCenter Clinic meets patients' needs while offering significant cost savings, and those savings are stretched further by innovative protocols that cut treatment time from several days in a hospital to one day of outpatient therapy. Proactive management of pain, side-effects, and hydration directly affect the need for hospitalizations of cancer patients. InfusiCenter nurses identify problems early and correct them before they become unmanageable and lead to a hospital admission.

The first InfusiCenter Clinic opened in Beverly Hills, California, in late 1988, and two more were opened patients by the end of 1989. Two others are in initial planning stages. The business plan calls for the clinics to be developed nationwide, and eventually Home Hospital Corporation plans to offer infusion therapy for narrowly defined groups, such as AIDS patients. The first clinics, however, are geared to oncology.

Cancer is a serious illness, but it is not necessarily fatal. One of three people with cancer survives. With some forms of the disease, nine of 10 people diagnosed eventually will be cured. Today, nearly 2 million Americans are considered cancer-free more than five years after initial diagnosis and treatment. A major reason for extended survival rates is rapid improvement of chemotherapy drugs, which physicians use in a substantial percentage of patients. Chemotherapy may be given orally, intramuscularly, or intravenously. Drugs that can irritate healthy tissue are best given in intravenous doses because blood flow helps dilute them. Many chemotherapy drugs given by IV are infused over a prolonged period to reduce toxic effects. Extra fluids may be infused to protect the kidneys, and other medications may be added to the chemotherapy regimen to counter-act side-effects such as nausea and vomiting. This complex treatment usually results in two to three days in a hospital.

In a hospital oncology unit, each nurse must care for many patients, and the individual patient receives only limited attention. Many patients find it traumatic to face a frightening ordeal in such an unfamiliar environment, and they have tremendous needs for personalized care.

The principles behind infusion therapy centers are not new. Twenty years ago all dialysis and even simple surgeries were inpatient procedures. But now community-based dialysis centers and outpatient surgicenters have transformed these treatments into almost exclusively outpatient procedures. We have applied the same model to infusion therapy.

Many cancer patients' first treatment experience is a physically and emotionally stressful inpatient surgical procedure. Afterward, one of the patient's first questions usually is whether he will have to return to the hospital for more treatment. The InfusiCenter Clinic allows physicians to offer a new answer that decreases stress and fosters the important self-visualization process. The patient can reason that if he does not need to be hospitalized again, perhaps his chances for complete recovery are good.

Patients need assurance that doctors and nurses will be attentive and responsive to their needs, and that confidence-building process starts before chemotherapy begins with the clinic's two to one staff-to-patient ratio. It is not uncommon for patients to visit the InfusiCenter Clinic in advance to see the infusion suite. This eases apprehension and allows visualization of the therapy.

The patients' personal introduction to InfusiCenter nurses is extremely important. In addition to administering chemotherapy, the nurses act as a primary source of information and emotional and family support, and that first visit links a caring face to the voice on the phone. This relationship makes the therapeutic process less intimidating and assures the patient that he will not undergo therapy alone. "I prayed to God for an angel to comfort me," said one patient. "Then my nurse Janet called me and explained the chemotherapy process, and I was not as afraid. Janet was with me during all my chemotherapy. She called me every day to see how I was feeling after I went home. My prayer was answered—Janet was my angel."

On the first visit, the nurse prepares the patient and family members and handles a barrage of questions. What time do I need to be there? What should I wear? Will I get sick? Can my spouse stay with me? The nurse gives all the answers and sends the patient home with a written agenda. The day before chemotherapy starts, the nurse calls the patient to answer more questions and offer reassurance. The next day, instead of greeting a stranger, the patient greets a person already known and trusted.

Coping with concerns about side-effects requires nurses to discuss digestive problems, nutrition, nausea and vomiting, mouth and throat problems, infection, hair loss, skin problems, and sexual dysfunction. Patients frequently ask questions or tell the nurse things that they are uncomfortable or embarrassed about discussing with the physician. They can handle these problems if they are prepared with accurate information in a caring and compassionate manner.

A typical patient will come to the center one day every month during the course of therapy. With arrival usually at about 9 a.m., the patient knows what to expect and, best of all, has already been introduced to the nurse. The patient is told to wear comfortable clothes and carry any personal items, such as tapes or books. Family members may stay nearby during the treatment.

Most chemotherapy regimens incorporate drugs that could cause renal toxicity, so the first few hours usually are devoted to intensive hydration. Patients may sit in comfortable recliners or stretch out on cozy beds as fluids are infused. The nurse closely monitors the intake and output of fluids to ascertain the appropriate balance and ensure that the kidneys are functioning properly. About 30 minutes prior to initiating the chemotherapy drugs, a series of medications are given to minimize the side effects—especially nausea and vomiting. Patients who undergo chemotherapy in this manner seldom experience nausea and vomiting, and that makes the process far more tolerable. Because these drugs are sedatives, patients typically sleep four to six hours after the drug is infused and hydration is resumed. During this therapy, the physician may visit the patient as often as necessary. The chart is easily accessible for monitoring clinical status, and the assigned nurse is always close at hand to answer questions.

When hydration is complete, the patient prepares to head home with clear instructions from the physician on recommended follow-up care. The patient must know what to expect after chemotherapy, such as continuing oral fluids at home and coping with side-effects. The patient will continue to ask the nurse a wide range of questions. The nurse can discuss frequency and duration of treatments, incidence and types of side effects, and medications to be taken at home. By 5 p.m., the patient has departed. Companions are required to drive because the patient is likely to feel drowsy.

Outpatient chemotherapy in the InfusiCenter Clinic offers many benefits. Patients spend less time away from home and can completely avoid an institutional environment. The chemotherapy experience is improved by the relaxed setting, the clinical expertise of the InfusiCenter nurses, and the emphasis on personal attention. Side-effects such as anticipatory nausea and vomiting are reduced. There is no risk of hospital-acquired infections. The InfusiCenter experience aids the success of therapy by improving patient compliance. Patients who have a negative experience with chemotherapy are more likely to discontinue therapy, thus decreasing their chances for cure.

Physicians appreciate the personalized clinical and emotional attention given to each patient. Because the nurse in the InfusiCenter clinic has fewer patients, more time is available for higher quality, one to one care. InfusiCenter Clinics generally are located in medical office buildings to make it convenient for referring physicians. They are pleased to be able to share in the comfortable environment as they visit patients during infusions—sometimes plopping into the recliner chair in the suite and relaxing with the patient.

InfusiCenter clinic nurses provide a daily written summary of therapy. Every follow-up phone call is documented and summarized for the physician. Follow-up notes and the therapy summary are in the chart, so the physician knows exactly how everything went and what issues the patient raised. This special attention to communication enhances care and saves the physician and his staff time and energy.

The InfusiCenter Clinic represents an exciting alternative for third-party payers. Outpatient infusion therapy costs them about half the expense of an average 2½-day, $2,000 to $3,000 hospital stay. Hospitalization accounts for the largest percentage of health care expenditures, and cancer patients often undergo multiple hospitalizations during the course of treatment. While insurers have experimented with many forms of cost containment with limited success, this innovation is worth exploring.

Medicare reimbursement remains low now, as is often the case when the government confronts an innovation. In fact, for some therapies, Medicare pays InfusiCenters less than the drugs cost. But Home Hospital Corporation is working on a demonstration project to show the federal government how it can save millions.

The InfusiCenter Clinic model has revolutionized the delivery of high acuity, complex infusion therapy. By challenging medical truisms about the "need" for hospitalization, the clinic idea will gain complete acceptance.

InfusiCenter Clinics will range in size from 1,200 to 3,000 square feet, with four to 10 beds. Clinics can be developed in medical office buildings with a minimum of special equipment, generally the high-tech pumps that control patient infusion rates. All administrative functions are handled at a central corporate office. InfusiCenter nurses must be highly trained in oncology and certified in chemotherapy to qualify for employment. After selection, they undergo an orientation program that thoroughly acquaints them with the InfusiCenter philosophy of care.

Physicians own InfusiCenter clinics, which are managed and developed by Home Hospital Corporation. Because the services are aimed at cancer patients, oncologists are the ideal physicians to involve as partners. To launch a successful clinic, three to six moderately busy oncologists are required, although this may vary with the type and volume of oncology practice. However, other specialists are not precluded from ownership, and large medical groups may succeed using the clinic for oncology and generalized infusion care. Physician groups that accept risk for the medical management of patients, such as independent practice associations, may enjoy a dual benefit by decreasing hospital expenditures and creating a new revenue source.

Home Hospital Corporation develops the center and operates it for the physician owners. The total cost of each new center is estimated at $200,000 to $300,000.

Hospital administrators usually view the clinic as direct competition at first, but a second look reveals benefits for the institution if the clinic is established as an outpatient department. The Medicare diagnosis related group for chemotherapy often is a money-loser for the hospital, but when this same procedure is performed in the InfusiCenter, it becomes a profitable treatment and frees a hospital bed for other kinds of patients. The main problem with hospital involvement with the InfusiCenter Clinic is the delay associated with institutional decision-making. Unfettered by bureaucracies, motivated physicians and medical groups can treat patients in their InfusiCenter clinic less than 60 days after agreements are signed.

———

PAUL SCHOLTES received his undergraduate education at Stanford University in human biology (A.B.), following which he completed a master of science in biology in a joint program with Stanford's department of biology and School of Medicine. After a second master of science degree in health services administration from a joint program with Stanford's schools of business and medicine, he received his law degree from the University of California, Berkeley, Boalt Hall School of Law. Mr. Scholtes has experience with HMOs and with home care services, and has been a featured speaker on home care issues for the California Association for Health Services at Home. He is chairman of the board and chief executive officer of InfusiCenter Clinics Group.

JULIA SHERMAN received her education at the University of the Pacific and the University of Arizona (B.S., Pharm.). She developed and directed the outpatient infusion clinic, home IV therapy, and nursing home care programs for Cigna Healthplans of Southern California. She currently is president of the InfusiCenter Clinics Group and Home Hospital Pharmacy, a division of Home Hospital Corporation. Ms. Sherman is a member of the American Society of Hospital Pharmacists and a Fellow of the American Society of Consultant Pharmacists.

Mr. Scholtes and Ms. Sherman are available to consult in their areas of expertise.

9

Developing and Managing
An Imaging Center

Cesar M. Mayo, M.D.

The development of magnetic resonance imaging (MRI) was one of the most significant events in the history of medical imaging. Without being invasive, MRI provides excellent ultrasensitive detection of lesions in the brain and spinal cord with no known biological hazards. Until the introduction of this new modality, computerized axial tomographic (CT) scanning was considered the gold standard of imaging. But with its excellent soft tissue definition, MRI has rapidly gained acceptance as the primary test for many central nervous system disorders.

MRI is not used to diagnose patients on life support, people who have suffered acute trauma, or those in whom early bleeding is suspected. But it already has replaced myelography as the principal study for spine and brain disorders, and it promises to supplant arthrography and arthroscopy in the investigation of musculoskeletal problems. MRI also holds promise for the imaging of other organ systems. In the future, three-dimensional image reconstruction and computerized image manipulation will become available, and we expect to use MRI angiography with simultaneous visualization of the arterial and venous circulation. We also anticipate manipulating images so that the plane of reference can be changed to suit the diagnostician's needs. Soon, scanner manufacturers will be upgrading their equipment to allow for dynamic examinations of joints in flexion and extension and motions of the spine and heart. Clearly we are seeing only the first hint of all the potential clinical applications of magnetic resonance imaging.

The brain has been the focus of initial investigation in most of the important developments in clinical imaging because no current device allows direct visualization of the central nervous system. An endoscope permits physicians to observe other organs and initiate treatments, but the brain has remained hidden and mysterious. Further, there are no reliable disease-specific biochemical tests for central nervous system function, and the brain and spinal cord do not permit the type of exploratory abdominal or thoracic surgery used when diagnostic tests fail to reveal definitive information. The usefulness of MRI to neurologists is clear.

Most imaging tests have started with studying the central nervous system. These include the use of opaque contrast material as employed in myelography and angiography. Indeed, the first angiogram was performed on the carotid artery. Similarly, ultrasound was first applied in the brain. We all remember when inferential diagnoses of space-occupying lesions in the brain were made by clearly demonstrating a shift of the "mid-line echo." Nuclear medicine and CT scans also had their start in the brain.

In 1984, I believed that MRI would become a vital medical tool whose use by physicians would grow dramatically as manufacturers perfected the technology and physicians applied it successfully, so I led the formation of a corporation owned by 32 physicians who invested in an MRI facility in San Jose. Over the next two years, the company expanded to two imaging centers with many other modalities, such as full x-ray service, ultrasound, mammography, nuclear medicine, and CT scanning. Along the way we learned a lot about the difficult task of entering into joint ventures with hospitals and obtaining third-party reimbursement for a service that was misunderstood by insurers and considered by some to be experimental.

Some physicians might be surprised to find a practicing clinical neurologist involved with imaging centers, but neurologists depend heavily on imaging studies. Colleagues in my specialty now stand at the forefront of diagnostic imaging ventures all over the United States. After the formation of the San Jose imaging centers, many clinical neurologists became involved with identical ventures elsewhere.

I heard the first serious discussion regarding the clinical applications of MRI in the brain in 1982. Even then, the images looked very good compared to CT images, but physicians had significant concerns that precluded the speedier introduction of MRI to clinical medicine. These included the magnet's size and weight, the excessive space requirements of adequate radiofrequency shielding, the extended length of the study, during which the patient often was required to be motionless, and the cost of the computer system. Except for its cost, most of these problems have been overcome. In fact, prices continue to escalate.

In 1983 I went to Pasadena, California, to visit a clinical facility that had gained substantial experience with magnetic brain imaging. I came away convinced that MRI was likely to replace CT scanning as the principal diagnostic test in the investigation of many central nervous system disorders.

My colleagues and I deliberated on the structure of the group and finally settled on a Subchapter S corporation. This has allowed us to send out a professional bill because each shareholder is a California licensed physician. This permitted the MRI center to bill for a global fee, including professional and facility charges, an advantage we continued to enjoy as we expand and offer other services. This also benefits Medicare patients because we accept assignment. It helped us sign contracts with preferred provider organizations and health maintenance organizations because we did not have to negotiate the professional component of the service separately.

The Subchapter S corporation allows tax benefits from initial losses to pass through to the owners. A major disadvantage is that S corporations cannot have more than 35 shareholders. This became a problem later, when many other physicians wanted to purchase shares. During the Christmas season of 1983, I contacted numerous San Jose area physicians about joining a new partnership that would develop and operate the San Jose Imaging Center.

Assuming that physicians with special interests in nervous system disorders would be most responsive, I personally contacted every neurosurgeon and neurologist from Santa Cruz to Livermore and from Palo Alto to Monterey. The response was mixed. Many shared my enthusiasm, but few were comfortable making a substantial investment in what was then an unproven and largely untested clinical imaging modality. MRIs had not been approved by the U.S. Food and Drug Administration. We approached hospitals, but administrators seemed uncomfortable with the imponderables brought on by the evolving system of Medicare diagnosis related group (DRG) reimbursements for inpatient care. They considered the project too risky because it had no track record of insurance reimbursement. With no other funding sources available other than physicians, we elected to expand the target physician group. I was certain MRI eventually would have many applications in diagnosis of cardiovascular disease, so we included internists and cardiologists. That did the trick. In only three weeks we had commitments from 32 physicians, mostly internists, to purchase 35 units of $21,500 each. About one-quarter of our investors were in neurological specialties.

Because the technology was so new, we had limited financing alternatives. There were no MRI equipment leasing firms then, so we had to go to a bank for a five-year loan. The note was secured completely by a prorated guarantee from each investor. I retained a medical management consulting firm that helped syndicate the group and served as a general contractor for our site in San Jose. This site is within one mile of a major hospital, two major freeways and a regional shopping center. We converted a 3,800-foot chiropractic office into the scanning center.

Because we were largely ignorant of the special design and construction requirements of an MRI center, we hired one of the nation's foremost MRI technologists from the radiation imaging laboratory of the University of California at San Francisco. At UCSF he had assisted in many of the world's first experimental MRI studies on animals and humans. His advice was immensely valuable as we constructed and installed our magnet and trained our first team of MRI technologists.

We created a physical plant that is warm, home-like, and not intimidating to patients. Services are competitively priced, and we offer discounts to HMOs and PPOs. We are proudest of our commitment to the elderly, which we demonstrate by accepting Medicare assignment. This alone has made us quite popular with seniors. The media reaction was very disappointing, however. Newspapers and television news departments were most interested in hyping the technology because it was so different and expensive. They did not care that a group of physicians had created an imaging center that offered a useful health care alternative at some financial risk.

We learned from our mistakes. The Subchapter S structure gives little control to the site manager. All direction is given by an operating board composed of busy practitioners who could not always give their full attention to management issues. They often could not attend entire board meetings, which were held every other week, even though we limited sessions to 90 minutes. With a wide-open agenda that could be distracted by any of them, the amount of productive guidance that emerged from the meetings was limited.

That led us to our situation today. We now contract with a management firm to run the imaging center. I head that company, reporting to the board at monthly meetings. My firm does all hiring and manages all aspects of the facility. When expertise is needed that I don't have, I hire consultants as necessary. This works more efficiently than consulting constantly with a hands-on board and gives management enough latitude to make necessary day-to-day decisions without decreasing its accountability to the investors.

When we opened our doors, our physician shareholders were obviously excited and enthusiastic. Others who had not become investors nonetheless were supportive, but a great majority of the medical community were skeptical. They had natural doubts about a free-standing site that would offer expensive, unproven technology in competition with accepted imaging modalities. As our loyal supporters promoted the technology and more people became convinced of its usefulness, the skeptics began referring patients. After about one year of operation, enough physicians were impressed with our apparent success to help us with the second round of financing.

As the business grew and it was apparent the MRI center was commercially viable, other financing options became available. We offered other physicians the chance to participate in an expanded imaging center at a second San Jose location one mile away. Expanding our investor base would help us battle encroaching competition. We chose subordinated participating notes as the means to launch the second phase. These seven-year notes are like bonds. They guarantee minimum 8-percent returns plus the potential for higher dividends depending on profitability. Since the second center opened, we have paid returns of about 20 percent, exceeding the minimum guaranteed to the investors.

Despite our success with physicians, I feel that limiting the investments to physicians is not desirable in view of increasing public sentiment against physician ownership of facilities they control and to which they refer patients. Public perceptions might improve if non-physicians, particularly local business people, were to purchase equal interests in such facilities.

After we had operated for a few months, I again approached area hospitals to offer them access to our technology. This time, I had a new concept. Because it was no longer possible for the hospitals to participate as shareholders, they could share this expensive and underused asset. We offered to scan patients in our facility and transmit digital MRI data by phone to computers inside each hospital. Films of studies could be generated in hospital radiology departments, thus giving radiologists the opportunity to read them and the hospital another service to market. But again we were frustrated by the hospitals' lack of interest.

Later we did succeed in entering into a joint venture with the for-profit arm of a non-profit hospital. The first stage was a 10-percent, $1.75-million loan to our center, with interest only due in the first year. This would give the hospital time to decide whether to stay with it over the long haul. We are now in the second stage of the joint venture, with a subordinated, participating debt similar to that of the physicians investors. The third stage will be the hospital's decision to convert the participating debt into equity or to withdraw from the venture. If the hospital elected to convert, the Subchapter S corporation would act as the general partner and the for-profit arm would become a limited partner.

There were numerous benefits to us in entering the joint venture with the hospital. It has improved medical staff relations. There is also the image of the hospital as having "deep pockets," which invariably encourages greater physician participation. The hospital can help obtain third-party contracts for our professional services. It has good contacts in the business and banking community that helped us obtain favorable bank loans. We also took advantage of the hospital's volume discounts on equipment acquisition. And finally, when the hospital joined us, the MRI center found increased public acceptance.

We started with great optimism but encountered serious problems dealing with the hospital in this joint venture. Every person involved in negotiating the relationship sensed that the hospital bureaucracy was slow and ambivalent about the partnership. Initially the hospital remained "competitive" with us, behaving as though every referral to the imaging center represented lost hospital revenue. This attitude was partly engendered by the fact that the for-profit arm profited from the venture at the expense of the hospital administration, which received no direct budgetary benefit from steering business to us. Unfortunately, because of internal factors and financial pressures at all their hospitals, the for-profit arm decided not to convert their debt into equity in our venture in 1990. Our MRI firm will continue to operate profitably as before, but we will go it alone.

As we fine-tuned our package of services in the first few years, we faced several regulatory problems. Because MRI was a new test that had not been approved for reimbursement by MediCal, California's Medicaid program, we had to lobby in Sacramento for the inclusion of MRI as a benefit. We ran into similar problems with worker's compensation carriers, which contended even after the Food and Drug Administration had approved MRI that the examination was experimental and not an accepted clinical tool. We took one of these carriers to court to fight that policy and in the process educated most of the others about the usefulness of MRI in the evaluation of back injuries and spine disorders. We thus paved the way for the reimbursement for MRI services by state worker's compensation carriers.

We encountered a "Catch-22" situation dealing with the substantial number of MediCal patients who were referred to our facility for various types of MRI studies. Many arrived late because they had transportation problems or they got lost. A few never showed up, and to smooth out these operating problems and maximize magnet utilization, I proposed a patient pickup and delivery service. I was prepared to use a well-equipped van that would come to the patient's residence, deliver him to the MRI facility for the study, and take him home afterward. On the way, the patient could watch a video that would explain the procedure and ease his anxiety.

We were all set to purchase the van when we ran into insurance difficulties. Insurance companies were unwilling to provide liability coverage for the van because it was involved in clinical services. Insurance brokers advised us that if we could obtain a letter from a state or local agency essentially requiring the MRI center to carry liability insurance on its patient transport van, they would be forced to write the coverage. We tried county, city, and state agencies but were unsuccessful in obtaining a regulation mandating insurance, so we abandoned this idea. This, of course, means that we had to continue to deal with the no-shows, cancellations without adequate notice, and inadequate reimbursement. This has been frustrating, but we have honored our pledge not to turn away people because of inability to pay. We continue to treat a substantial number of MediCal patients despite extremely low MediCal reimbursement.

Appropriateness of care issues can be difficult because utilization reviewers have few established guidelines regarding MRIs. The problem centers on the paucity of information received by the imaging center about the indications for the study. In a hospital, the patient's chart can settle questions. But that information does not always reach the outpatient establishment. Because it is a new technology, the real concern is whether the test is justified. Initially, we made the radiologist the final arbiter of whether a study is needed. Based on information about the patient, which sometimes necessitated a phone call to the referring physician, the radiologist could decide whether the MRI or an alternative exam might be more useful. The radiologist has no personal financial incentive to maximize MRI utilization.

Educational programs always enhance services, so I encouraged and assisted our first MRI radiologist in developing a training program for physicians. Because MRI was new and in great demand, our radiologist established fellowships lasting six months to a year, which we funded with assistance from the magnet vendor. We wanted our facility to become one of the premier imaging centers in the nation. After that time, each fellow felt supremely confident in his ability to understand the technology and direct an MRI facility. We hosted one-week visiting fellowships, during which trainees received many hours of didactic instruction interspersed with hands-on exposure and clinical interpretation. They also completed personal reviews of an extensive teaching file. These visiting fellowships became quite popular in our first two years, and our on-site radiologist developed a national reputation. Applications flowed in from all over the country and some foreign nations. We also ran a training program for MRI technologists. Most technologists, even those with extensive CT experience, cannot simply switch to MRI work after one week of training, which is the maximum offered by most MRI vendors. At our sites, we require at least three months' training, and even those who had completed this formal program were supervised for at least three additional months.

Because MRI technology was new and clinical experience at most sites was limited, we were concerned about liability. We established careful patient selection criteria and kept in close contact with the UCSF radiology department and the scanner manufacturer about MRI indications and contraindications. Initially, a radiologist would personally interview every patient. We were cautious about dealing with the acutely ill, and we refused to scan patients with an unstable cardiovascular status. We required a physician to remain on the premises at all times during scanning.

It became evident early in our experience that MRI is useful in evaluating AIDS patients because of its capacity to identify disseminated lesions in the brain. To allay concerns of technologists and other patients about exposure to human immunodeficiency virus, we established guidelines on handling of AIDS patients. Throughout the scanning process we maintain visual and intercom contact, and, if necessary, post one or two individuals in the scanning room. All employees are certified for basic life support, and we established close relations with the local ambulance company to assure its rapid response time if we ever need to rush a patient back to the hospital.

Despite the precautions, we had an unfortunate experience that should serve as a cautionary tale for all MRI facility operators. We performed a scan on a patient who had an undetected metal fragment embedded in his eye. The patient, a former iron worker who was referred to us by a military facility, was acutely ill from a blood disorder and was almost terminal. While the study was under way, he complained of eye pain and said he could not see. Apparently the powerful magnet torqued the metal fragment out of place and caused a large vitreous hemorrhage. He subsequently went blind. Because of this incident, every MRI facility in the world invariably asks if the patient has a metallic foreign body in the eye or has ever been employed as an iron worker.

The project was well-conceived and executed, but we physicians quickly realized we were in over our heads when it came to business and financial matters. We made up for this by hiring competent business people. We strived to obtain the highest caliber of professional services and contracted with the O'Connor Hospital group of radiologists. We have professional marketing assistance and high-quality accounting service. We recruited a good staff of technologists dedicated to patient care and customer satisfaction. We bought state-of-the-art equipment and introduced new services to the community, first with MRI, most recently with single photon emission computed tomography (SPECT), a nuclear medicine procedure that allows us to measure gamma emission from injected isotopes. The increased sensitivity of the SPECT technique permits us to acquire more precise images showing metastatic cancer in bone and other organs and earlier signs of tissue injury in the brain and heart caused by vascular disease. We remain at the leading edge of scanning technologies.

Physicians now use MRI to obtain early and accurate diagnosis of many clinical problems, improve therapeutic planning (as in the staging of malignancies) and perform mapping of surgical procedures. For example, orthopedic surgeons can see the soft-tissue extension of tumors and avoid disarticulation or extensive amputation of limbs in patients with bone cancer affecting the extremities. Through a wide excision, complete tumor removal is possible. Because of its ability to offer images in several planes, MRI also helps oncologists plan radiation therapy.

For patients, our MRI center has eliminated some expensive and painful invasive tests, reduced anxiety, and offered predictable, convenient outpatient diagnostic studies. The smells, sounds, and sights of the hospital, with its acutely ill patients, are gone. The service costs less because of lower outpatient facility overhead, and the benefits of improved care and physician planning flow directly to the patients. Payers take advantage of competitive local pricing structures, improved quality that allows earlier diagnosis, prompt treatment, and avoidance of inpatient days for diagnostic purposes. The litany of benefits makes it clear: The MRI center concept is here to stay and could be replicated anywhere with as much benefit to the community and investors as we have seen in San Jose.

CESAR M. MAYO, M.D., received his undergraduate and medical education at the University of Santo Tomas, Manila, Philippines. After an internship at U.S. Air Force Hospital, Clark Air Force Base, Pampanga, Philippines, he served one year of internal medicine and neurology residency at Santo Tomas University Hospital. He completed neurology residency training at the University of Louisville Hospitals, Louisville, Kentucky, and the Detroit Receiving Hospital, Detroit. He completed his chief residency in neurology at the University of Louisville Hospitals. A two-year fellowship in neuropathology followed at Northwestern University Medical School, Evanston, Illinois. Dr. Mayo remained on the faculty at Northwestern University Medical School in the department of neurology from 1964 to 1969. He then accepted a faculty position as assistant professor of neurology at Albany Medical College, Albany, New York, in 1969, and the following year was named associate professor. In 1971 he became chief of the neurology service, Veterans Administration Hospital, Martinez, California. Dr. Mayo is a Diplomate of the American Board of Psychiatry and Neurology, as well as the American Board of Electrodiagnostic Medicine. He is a Fellow of the American College of Physicians, the American Academy of Neurology, and the American Geriatric Society. He is founder and president of the San Jose Imaging Center and Pacific Imaging Services, Inc. Dr. Mayo is available as a consultant in the area of imaging center development.

10

Starting a Multispecialty Clinic

Peter Crandall, M.D.

During the many years in which I ran a successful OB-GYN solo practice in San Jose, California, I never expected to wind up in a multispecialty group medical practice. But the profound changes in the health care delivery system that took root at the beginning of the 1980s brought about significant new advantages to those who choose to work in large group settings. A group has far more leverage than an individual when purchasing equipment and supplies or when negotiating contracts with insurance companies. The strength of a group's relationship with a hospital exceeds that of a solo physician, and a group is better able to enter into joint ventures with outpatient facilities. Patients prefer the "one-stop shopping" of a group practice. And, finally, but not unimportantly, the camaraderie that develops among physicians when practicing with others is a major benefit.

The task of assembling a large multispecialty group practice is a demanding and sometimes maddening experience involving an avalanche of details and decisions. Success requires the group to be simultaneously prudent and opportunistic, able to react to changes quickly in order to position itself for the future. The Good Samaritan Medical Group originated in 1981, when Dr. Fred Armstrong, an internist, felt the time was right for a multispecialty group practice in the San Jose area. The rise of managed care called for group contracts, and San Jose was home to a glut of independent physicians and an undersupply of multispecialty groups. With change comes opportunity, he said, and Good

Samaritan seemed to be a good one. Dr. Armstrong invited local physicians to a discussion of the idea. The first meeting drew approximately 40 physicians, each of whom was asked to contribute $100 to cover expenses. Nearly everyone wrote a check, including me.

The physicians who attended our meeting later were asked to put up a refundable $1,000 investment, and the field immediately narrowed to about 20 physicians. The winnowing process continued with a request for another $5,000 per doctor, a sum that separated the committed physicians from everyone else. We had five internists and one obstetrician. The American Medical Association once projected that the number of practices with more than 150 physicians might reach 250 by 1995, and we all wondered whether Good Samaritan might be one of them.

Despite our small size, the medical community did not perceive us as elitist or exclusive. Dr. Armstrong had invited a large number of local physicians to join. Those who didn't join knew that they were not excluded. It was their own decision. This simple fact has neutralized any feelings of fear or jealousy that would otherwise be expected from neighboring physicians. The six core physicians were firmly committed to the plan, and in some ways the small size of the group made the organizational process easier. We felt we could build a fair financial structure faster with six participants than with many more. But even with only six, it became clear that little would be accomplished without authentic leadership. There are as many ideas as there are people, and everyone must be allowed to express his or her views. The leaders had to allow physicians to ventilate, and, while it sometimes seemed as if we were accomplishing very little, some physicians did take charge and keep the group moving forward. The key was to distill everyone's thoughts so they weren't repeated needlessly. We used an easel to record notes of every motion or piece of relevant information and to keep the group from wasting precious time by re-hashing points.

It has been eight years since those first exploratory sessions—three years of planning and five years of hard work with meetings every Monday night at 6 p.m. Many of these sessions lasted until midnight. We still are absolutely amazed at the number of details that must be studied and weighed to assure that every decision is fair and beneficial to all group members. Lopsided decisions that fail to account for all viewpoints can lead to hard feelings, and we learned that these conflicts simply must be talked out to keep them from creating needless friction. We surveyed ourselves and found that our physicians possessed expertise in a variety of areas, including mathematics, computers, electronics, politics, and health insurance. Our extracurricular capabilities certainly didn't even come close to covering all our needs, but we were able to adapt a program that played to our individual strengths.

We brought the lawyers to the table and developed the articles of incorporation, bylaws, buy/sell provisions, and income-distribution formulas. The corporation was born and named three years before we welcomed the first patient into the group office. The income distribution formula became a major concern because there were considerable disparities among the physicians' independent incomes. We set down fair principles and built a compensation program around them. The earnings distribution had to resemble the specialty variations seen in private practice. Because we were a group, some income sharing would be necessary, and so everyone agreed to contribute five percent of their individual incomes to a fund that would be apportioned equally to all members. We devised specialty factors that increased a physician's contribution to the fund based on how many standard deviations his current income was from the norm. The greater that variance, the more money the physician would contribute to the pot for equal redistribution. But at the same time, we agreed that the entire physician compensation plan must be incentive-driven, and the group limited how much could be channeled into that fund to prevent the formula from functioning as a disincentive. Finally, we had to derive a fair formula for cost accounting. When we were marketing to bring in additional physicians, we had even greater variations among physician incomes and physician need of floor space. The cost-accounting formula allowed for allocations of expenses based on areas occupied by the physicians. The formula seemed to work very well, but it must be noted that it was a cash-oriented formula, based on collections. Because a new corporation has no revenue, the formula could not be used readily, although portions of it were immediately applicable. We decided to pay everyone an overhead base to keep incomes proportional to amounts earned previously.

We all continued to work in our private practices during the organizing phase, so our accounts receivable generated enough cash flow to enable us to make loans to the new group as part of our investment. The physicians' salaries were continued from the old accounts receivable in the individual offices, and when needed, advances were made from our line of credit. One should note that the Internal Revenue Service does not permit commingling of funds from the two practices, so separate accounting systems had to be maintained.

To build the group into a full-fledged multispecialty practice, we sought physicians we thought would fit our corporate culture. We already knew the quality of their work from years of association in medical societies, insurance organizations, and professional review organizations. We looked at the style of their practice. All this information was helpful, but one insight often outweighed all the background data we could gather on a physician. If a candidate asked, "What can you do for me?" we knew he would not be a team player. The ones who asked, "What can I do for the group?" turned out to be excellent members. That has been true of every physician we have brought into the organization since the original six joined forces.

Shortly after we started the planning process, we expanded the group to 13 physicians, and on moving day we had two obstetricians, four pediatricians and seven internists. Six months later, a general practitioner, a surgeon, a urologist and an ear, nose and throat specialist joined us. The second year, we added an orthopedic surgeon, two obstetricians, another pediatrician, and a dermatologist. Today the group has 25 physicians, and we're conscious of the need not to grow too rapidly. To help us avoid taking on any sub-specialist before we have enough patients to keep him busy, we consider published guidelines on how many patients are necessary to support a practitioner in that particular specialty.

We had no expertise in dealing with a bank. At the beginning, we established a $250,000 line of credit, but this quickly proved woefully inadequate. The cash flow of a brand new corporation is severely limited, so the line of credit must be large. Like any start-up company, a medical group has a severe shortage of cash while developing its product and getting it to the marketplace. Debt service cannot start until the product is for sale and the cash starts to stream into the business. Because a new corporation has no track record, banks are very reluctant to provide major funding. As our business took off, the banks became more interested. Today we have good banking relationships, but anyone building a new medical group should find a manager with extensive knowledge of the banking industry.

We wanted ample room for growth, but it would be prohibitively expensive to lease extra space for the future. We found a medical office developer that planned to construct a 35,000-square-foot building. The landlord was willing to lease the group 12,000 square feet, of which we would immediately occupy 9,000. But when the time came to install the partitions, we directed the developer to finish the entire 12,000 square feet and we purchased an option on another 6,000 square feet. Today we occupy all of that space and have added a new medical records room, a business office, a laboratory, and three nonadjacent locations within the medical office complex—a total of 28,000 square feet. We are committed to a staff-to-MD ratio of 3 to 1 and currently have 72 full-time positions. We placed all staff members in the front area where they could assist each other and interact with the rest of the employees in the warmly decorated environment. The group had to purchase new waiting room chairs and other furnishings. We were able to use most of the equipment we had brought into the practice from our previous offices, although some of it had to be repainted or reupholstered. Now, in our third year, we have no more room for expansion. The only way to squeeze more value out of the existing space is to lengthen the hours of operation with a second shift of employees and physicians, a move that would effectively double the space.

A large group practice requires sophisticated accounting. We decided to automate the accounting department and also assumed that we would need computer capabilities for all patient charting. The computer we bought would have to be large enough to handle it all. But after looking at four or five different systems, we approached the question from the standpoint of hardware reliability and asked the hardware vendors to identify the best software people. Group members made site visits to determine how user-friendly the software was and what its users thought of it. We ultimately selected Hewlett-Packard hardware and Psi-Med software. This decision has benefited the group during the initial rapid growth phase because we were able to retain the same software through the increasingly larger Hewlett-Packard systems without having to manipulate the data for each system revision. During our hectic short-term growth period, this has been a marvelous advantage.

The amount of data storage needed for a medical group is staggering. We started with a capacity of 135 megabytes—about 135 million characters and other bits of data—but were only able to fit half our data in that space. We wound up adding 404 megabytes of capacity. Then, as the physician roster grew longer, we ran out of capacity for additional terminals and printers, and that required us to obtain another computer. Of course, with each physician comes hundreds or thousands of additional patients, so we had to buy a third computer that increased our ports from 12 to more than 150. With the client base currently at 70,000 patients, payment mechanisms have become increasingly varied. Some patients are capitated health maintenance organization members, others have an HMO fee-for-service system with no balance billing, some are preferred provider organization members with fee-for-service discounts, some are regulated by Medicare and Medicaid, and others continue using traditional insurance programs. Each category has subtle billing nuances related to copayments, balance billing, and discounts, and all those factors must be integrated into accounting and reporting functions that provide useful information on our financial performance.

The keyboard entry of the physicians' patient databases became a major project. The accounts receivable and clinical information were drawn from files in nine different medical offices. We had to set up the computer months in advance and have the office staff translate handwritten ledger cards into meaningful information in the computers. Imagine for a moment a new computer brought on-line with software unknown to anybody in nine offices. The staffs had to be trained in short order to enter the data and understand the software. They were asked to perform the work after hours, at lunchtime, or before their offices opened in the morning. It was mass confusion! Eventually the group hired a consulting firm to straighten out mistakes we made involving patients' addresses and family relationships.

The telephone system is a pivotal part of the business. In deciding whether to lease or buy, we had to learn how many telephone lines and calls we would need. To our surprise, we found significant differences in telephone computer switches. We ended up spending $85,000 on the communications system.

For patient charting, we chose a numeric system over an alphabetic system so the computer could track accounts and files more efficiently. The group hired a medical records librarian to integrate the chart system, a task that was far more complex than anticipated. Planning the size of a chart room also was very difficult. In our worst miscalculation, we estimated we would have 300 chart-pulls a day. We actually wound up with 900 chart-pulls a day while still in our infancy. The histories and physicals were found to be totally different at the various offices, and all the alphabetic charts had to be converted to new jackets. The group started with a movable aisle charting system, but it proved to be grossly inadequate, and we replaced it with an open stack system. Now our system can accommodate up to 40 physicians at the main office. Our old charts have been transferred to a storage system that can retrieve any record in 24 hours.

We looked at conveyor belts, pneumatic tubes, and dumbwaiters when selecting a chart transport system. We chose one of the many available pneumatic tubes for delivering one chart at a time in response to a phone call, as opposed to bringing in all the charts expected for that day's service.

As we moved into the building, we had conferred with pathologists and radiologists about creating joint ventures for our laboratory and x-ray departments. We now have a management contract for the radiology department. Our laboratory has worked out well except for our lack of space. The volume of patients going through the laboratory at times can be overwhelming. The radiology joint venture has been satisfactory, but we had to set it up in a location about 100 yards from our main office. Patients occasionally object to the distance, but for the most part it has been satisfactory.

We decided early in the group's history to find an administrative manager, but we did not have the money to put one on the payroll just then. Until we were ready, a consultant helped keep us organized. The interview process to hire a manager was time-consuming. We ran newspaper advertisements, sorted through résumés, and narrowed a large number of applicants down to 10 people for interviews. We sought a manager able to listen to all the physicians, treat them all fairly, hire and fire the support staff, and find new accounting systems and accountants. The position required a confident individual who was not quite so headstrong that he would not adhere to the concepts developed by the group's board.

The managerial challenge of merging nine medical office staffs into a single corporation cannot be overstated. One unit may be a group of three pediatricians and their loyal staff, while another might be a solo obstetrician and his or her staff. Each had similar needs but different points of view. Some of the personnel on the amalgamated staff were too strong for the group, and others were better suited to smaller medical offices. As the myriad personalities interacted and such strengths and weaknesses became apparent, a kind of natural selection occurred, with people joining and leaving the staff over time. After three years, some office staff members still maintain allegiance to the physician who brought them on board, but creation of personnel protocols and employee handbooks with formal policies have erased many of the inconsistencies. Many more people have been hired since then, and different departments have been brought together more effectively. But the problems were by no means limited to the office staff. Physicians also could be very difficult to work with. They had strong feelings about how they previously had done their charting and bookkeeping, and some were not willing to give up their familiar habits when everything else was being changed around them.

Before the group opened its doors, the nine offices had nine different accountants that worked for their clients. But the group had to settle on a single accountant. We conducted interviews and made a choice. Since then, it has become apparent that the best accounting firm for a group of this size is one that can deal with complex financial computer systems, handle legal aspects of accounting issues, perform tax planning, and develop accounting systems.

Our crystal ball says that groups are the strongest players and that networking and consolidation of groups is the way of the future. With new employees in the business office to neutralize obsolete loyalties to individual bosses, good management, close attention to cash flow, and preservation of democratic decision-making processes, groups can offer physicians a cooperative working environment and professional security during the 1990s —a decade that promises to be an era of rapid change in medicine.

PETER CRANDALL, M.D., received his undergraduate education at San Jose State College (B.A., Chemistry), and his medical education at George Washington University Medical School, Washington, D.C. (M.D., 1962). After a rotating internship at San Francisco General Hospital, he served a four-year residency in obstetrics and gynecology at the University of Oregon Medical School Hospitals, Portland, Oregon, and then served as chief of OB-GYN service, Holloman Air Force Base, New Mexico. He entered private practice in San Jose, California, and has been active in numerous professional societies and groups. He is a founding member and past president of the Good Samaritan Medical Group, former president of the Santa Clara County Foundation for Medical Care, and a member of the board of directors of Lifeguard HMO. Dr. Crandall is a Diplomate of the American Board of Obstetrics and Gynecology and a Fellow of the American College of Obstetrics and Gynecology. He is active in the Rotary Club of Saratoga, California. He is available to consult in the area of multispecialty clinic development.

11

Recovery Care Centers

Tony Carr, B.A., M.S.

During my indoctrination as a hospital administrator years ago, a prominent Princeton University health care economist built an entire philosophy on the assumption that the hospital was the center of the health care universe and all health care services radiated from it like the spokes of a wheel. The changes in health care since then have been profound and rapid, and such ideas seem almost charming now. In 1969, the East Coast medical establishment was appalled by reports of how "charlatan anesthesiologists" in Phoenix opened the first free-standing surgery center. At first, outpatient surgery grew slowly. In 1980, only 15 percent of surgery in the central California community of Fresno was performed in the outpatient setting. But by 1986, more than 50 percent of Fresno's surgery was done on an outpatient basis. We may see similar progress in another revolutionary health care movement thanks to a new California law that establishes a network of post-surgical recovery care centers.

A major challenge to medicine is to admit the patient to the most appropriate level of care and then discharge the patient as soon as possible. The post-surgical recovery care center helps accomplish this goal. This new facility is a special hospital designed for healthy Class I and Class II patients who require an overnight environment of general nursing care and pain control for 24 to 72 hours. This is a new level of acute care.

A recent headline in Modern Healthcare magazine said, "At Last, a Cure for Wellness." That sums up the recovery care center movement, which will spread across the country with a new level of care for healthy patients who do not need the complex technological services of an acute care hospital. For too long, these patients have been paying for hospital services they don't need or use. The average length of stay for patients at the recovery care center is significantly shorter than in hospitals. For example, non-Medicare patients undergoing cholecystectomy in a hospital have an average length of stay of 4.5 days. In our facility, that is cut to 2.2 days.

The Fresno Surgery Center was founded by general partner Dr. Alan H. Pierrot, who launched it in 1984 with 95 physician limited partners. It has five operating rooms and two treatment rooms. At about that time, a leading orthopedic surgeon in Fresno lamented that if only he could keep his patients in the surgery center for 24 or 48 hours, he could eliminate his hospital practice. As a result of that discussion, we decided to poll physicians on our staff to learn what other types of patients might require only 24 to 48 hours of nursing care, IV fluids, and pain control. Not surprisingly, we found that this pool of patients represented a larger segment of the market than anyone initially envisioned. By surveying four community hospitals, we found that 35 to 40 percent of in-hospital surgery qualified for a recovery care facility.

Because of the positive response from that poll, we decided to explore a licensing waiver from the state of California that would permit us to provide this service. We contacted a government relations consulting firm that represents surgery centers to see if we could take advantage of skilled nursing facility regulations that allow for "program flexibility." The bureaucrats were interested in our innovation, but the issue was too volatile for them to handle administratively. They didn't want to touch it. We opted to take the legislative route. So we drafted legislation that would modify the state's existing skilled nursing facility standards and carved away those guidelines that relate primarily to the geriatric component of skilled nursing care. We sought an environment to care for healthy patients who need pain control and nursing care on an overnight basis. When the legislation was introduced in March, 1986, it caught the hospitals by surprise.

The state hospital association tracks legislation using a computer that screens new bills for certain key words. None of those words were in our bill, so when we went to a legislative hearing, we were amazed to find absolutely no opposition. With the backing of state Sen. Kenneth Maddy, a Republican from the San Joaquin Valley, the bill cleared the Senate Health Committee without opposition. In essence, the original proposed legislation called for a new type of care that modified existing skilled nursing facility standards for appropriately screened post-surgical patients.

The hospital association eventually woke up and recognized the ramifications of our new level of care. Most of the opposition's arguments against our proposal were the same as those used by detractors of ambulatory surgery facilities more than a decade earlier. The hospital association accused our physicians of trying to line their pockets by competing with nonprofit community hospitals. We were told recovery care facilities would skim the profitable cases, leaving only the complex surgical cases and the charity care in the hospital. I found this odd because I was taught during my training that hospitals were for sick people, and that our goal was to get people out of the hospital. The association said that high-overhead hospitals were not positioned to compete with recovery care centers for healthy patients, and that was true. The hospitals' costs would increase because healthy patients would shift to this new level of care. But the hospitals failed to consider that employers wanted relief from rising health costs.

The hospital association circulated "code blue" bulletins to more than 600 California hospitals, warning them that our bill would partition the patient population the way ambulatory surgery centers snared healthy patients who could have surgery outside the hospital. This, they claimed, would bump traditional outpatients into an overnight environment, thereby making more money for the greedy physicians. And they warned that recovery care centers would compromise quality because patient safety would be sacrificed.

But the legislators recognized the hospitals' political barrage for what it was: fear of competition. The lawmakers saw beyond the hospital association's parochial interests and believed that recovery care centers would emerge as a new level of service that would provide inpatient care at significantly lower cost than acute care hospitals. After the dust settled, strong legislation passed, albeit with some compromises. Although some provisions of the legislation are not logical, such as the 72-hour limit on patient stays, we are living with it for the moment. We did achieve 80 percent of our goals. Signed in September, 1986, the law:

• Required the creation of 12 demonstration projects within a three-year pilot program. This compromise forced our industry to move slowly in order to prove the validity of the recovery care facility concept and the appropriateness of the patient selection process.

• Defined the facilities as separate and free-standing. Even though hospitals and nursing homes can establish recovery care centers without this legislation, the thrust of the legislation was to create truly free-standing facilities, independent of hospitals.

• Restricted the length of stay to 72 hours and defined eligible patients as those needing 24 to 48 hours of care. If a third night were necessary, approval for that extended stay would have to be made by the attending physician and the recovery care center medical director.

• Limited the number of beds to 20 per center. Originally, our intent was to build 16 beds within our free-standing surgery center, so this restriction was not seen as a sacrifice.

The California Office of Statewide Health Planning implemented the law with the help of a technical advisory committee that oversees the development of standards of care for patients and construction guidelines. These standards have been a hybrid of existing skilled nursing facility and acute care hospital standards. I believe the new standards have considerable flexibility because the state wants this program to work. I was impressed with the way the state handled implementation.

The pilot program will permit three types of recovery care centers. First is a recovery care center attached to an existing free-standing surgery center, which is the model we adopted. Fortunately, our surgery center is in a professional office park that could accommodate a recovery care center annex, allowing an integrated program. The second type allows the recovery care center operating within a skilled nursing facility or acute care hospital. The third type is a free-standing center that receives post-surgical patients from hospitals or free-standing surgery centers via ambulance. The proposed regulation limits the distance between those feeder facilities and the recovery center to 15 miles.

The demonstration project has been extended to 1994. Most facilities will either be separate and free-standing or attached to a surgery center.

As part of our initial marketing survey in Fresno, we asked physicians to suggest the types of surgical patients who would appropriately be admitted to a recovery care center. The list of surgical procedures was quite long and included ligament repairs, knee or shoulder reconstruction, mastectomy and mammoplasty, hemorrhoidectomy, nasal septoplasty, transurethral prostatectomy, thyroidectomy, vaginal hysterectomy, cholecystectomy, and many other surgical procedures. Several neurosurgeons also are interested in admitting patients following microlaminectomies.

From our review of inpatient surgical schedules at four community hospitals, we estimate that 35 to 40 percent of current inpatient surgical cases would be appropriate for recovery care. In our community of about 500,000, we projected a total market of about 5,000 cases appropriate for admission to our facility, and our goal became a market penetration of 25 to 30 percent, or 1,000 to 1,500 cases a year. With the recovery care center next to the surgicenter, we saw an opportunity to increase our share of the outpatient surgery market by offering more convenience. A surgeon can now manage outpatients and recovery care patients at the same location. We were motivated to act aggressively because area hospitals had signed exclusive contracts with health maintenance organizations, denying us a significant segment of the market. We had to do something.

We hired a major accounting firm to test our assumptions and evaluate the feasibility of this new venture. We asked the accountants to determine actual costs for patients we could admit to the recovery care center. They showed that the average charge for a cholecystectomy in the hospital was $5,000, whereas our charge for the same patient, including the surgicenter fee, would be $2,300—a savings to the patient of 54 percent. A thyroidectomy would cost 43 percent less at a recovery care center; hemorrhoidectomy, 29 percent; mastectomy, 56 percent; ligament repair, 29 percent; rotator cuff repair, 45 percent. The projected overall average savings was about 30 percent.

The potential savings in health care costs was a major factor that made this bill attractive to the state legislators. If we can offer such substantial savings, hospitals will be forced to reduce their charges. It has happened before. When we opened our surgery center in 1984, the largest hospital in town reduced its outpatient surgery charges by 30 percent. Yet the hospital charges still remained higher than ours.

It took two years for the Office of Statewide Health Planning to develop standards and for us to build the Fresno Recovery Care Center adjacent to our surgicenter. We opened in September, 1988, with 20 private rooms, 10 each on the second and third floors. Because we are small, we can maintain a warm and friendly environment. Just as we have seen with surgery centers, we are committed to patient care and comfort. With only 20 beds, a recovery care center can serve more than 2,500 patients a year.

We don't want people to feel they are in an acute care hospital, so we created a residential and hotel ambience with a warm and calming decor. On the first floor we have a conference room, kitchen, endoscopy suite, and lobby. Recovery care patients and outpatients register in the waiting room of the surgery center. If patients leave the recovery care center saying it wasn't like a hospital at all, we feel complimented. We want the facility to reflect excellence, quality, and concern for patients and visitors. We strive to provide an environment that does not disrupt families or friendships.

The health industry has neglected privacy for too long. Most patients want their doors closed, so each room is private and larger than the semi-private rooms in most community hospitals.

If the patient is comfortable and relaxed, healing is hastened and the length of stay reduced. Each room has a sofabed, and we encourage family members to stay overnight with patients and help in their recovery. If rooming-in is good for kids in pediatric hospitals, it is good for adults too. About 40 percent of the patients have a family member stay overnight with them. Complimentary meals are offered to family members. We have determined that food is actually one of the cheapest yet most appreciated services we can provide. Good food is important to patients' sense of well-being even though they may not eat very much. We also send the chef into the patients' rooms to determine special likes and dislikes.

The rooms are equipped with mini-bars, VCRs, and the largest televisions of any hospital in town. The rooms have four speakers for the radio and television, and patients have access to a video movie library. In addition we have many interesting books available for patients and families to enjoy.

We support local artists and have purchased 100 pieces of original art for display in patient rooms and throughout the facility. We use the art to camouflage some of the medical functions in the rooms. The oxygen and suction outlets are hidden behind paintings that are mounted on hinges and swing out for easy access. Each room also comes with a terry cloth bathrobe and a built-in hair dryer.

On each floor are many places for private consultations between physicians and families. Although the state wouldn't permit a fireplace, we built an ersatz model so we could have a mantel in the lobby. The nursing station on each floor is pivotal. Rather than being tucked off in a corner, we designed it so people would feel comfortable going to it. By dramatically increasing the width of the corridor to 18 feet, we created a lobby-like effect around it.

During 1989, we served 767 adult and pediatric patients. Although the pilot program allows us to care for children over age one, there is a pediatric hospital in the community, and consequently we do not see many small children. We do admit many school-age children, particularly those with athletic injuries. Our average length of stay has remained steady at two days, and the average charge for surgery and overnight care now stands at about $2,900.

The two most frequently performed procedures have been ligament repairs and cholecystectomies. The program is excellent for treating breast cancer. You can provide the biopsy, the mastectomy, and breast reconstruction in a soothing, comfortable environment.

The orthopedic surgeons have been the driving force behind the development of the Recovery Care Center. About 35 percent of our admissions have been orthopedic, 20 percent general surgery, and the remainder gynecological, ear, nose, and throat, plastic, and urological surgery. I project that in the near future orthopedics and gynecology will be about equal in volume as we do more hysterectomies. The results for women who have had hysterectomies have been excellent.

In our first 18 months, we have transferred only one patient to a hospital because she had already been under our care for the maximum 72 hours. Twenty percent of our patients stayed beyond two days. The demonstration program requires the physicians to provide details for the patient record whenever a patient stays longer than 48 hours, although we believe this burden doesn't make sense. In 1989, we averaged 66 patients a month. The busiest month so far has seen 80 patients admitted to the recovery care center. We view our break-even as being about 60 patients a month, and that assumes we continue serving 20 surgical outpatients a day.

We are convinced that 70 percent of all surgery is appropriate for outpatient or recovery care environments, and that is probably conservative. In Fresno in 1986, for the first time ever, more surgical procedures were performed on an outpatient basis than in hospitals— about 55 percent versus 45 percent. The American Hospital Association recently predicted that about 60 percent of all surgery would be performed on an outpatient basis by 1995. When combined with those surgical procedures which, because of recovery care centers, can now be moved to the outpatient area, a very large segment of the surgical population never will see the inside of an acute care hospital. In 10 years, perhaps we will be talking about 90 percent. If we dream beyond the way we do things now, as we move toward more non-invasive ways of treating patients, new surgical procedures, and improvements in anesthesia, someday I'll rent a billboard in Fresno and offer nausea-free surgery and postoperative care without the hazards of an acute care hospital.

In order to provide the best in nursing care, we employ only registered nurses. I wish someone could determine how to measure the quality impact of a staff composed entirely of RNs. I wouldn't do it any other way, because this is the way nursing was meant to be practiced. Because of the superior working conditions, we have had no difficulty recruiting nurses. We have a minimum of two nurses per 10 beds. Our detractors accuse us of not providing a safe environment, but all our RNs are certified for advanced cardiac life support. The staffing ratio is higher than in a hospital, and the nursing hours per patient day are significantly greater. The payoff comes in more comfort and a reduced length of stay. Patient evaluations have been outstanding, with 98 percent stating they would choose the recovery care center again and 100 percent saying they would recommend us to friends and relatives.

Our center uses the latest patient-controlled analgesic units for postoperative pain management—another service we can promote for healthy patients. Our orientation is wellness, and this makes a world of difference. So far our nosocomial infection rate is zero. We plan further surveillance to understand why this is so, but we won't delay in publicizing this as an advantage of recovery care.

Hospitals have retaliated by taking some of our surgeons' block time away and emphasizing in their commercials that they have medical back-up, which implies that we don't. We hear accusations that we are skimming the cream, bumping outpatients up to inpatient status, and compromising on quality care. But the common thread in all the attacks is the competition that we represent. The irony is that in the future, hospitals could become the major providers of recovery care.

Anyone who wants to start a recovery care center should bear in mind that Medicare approval is vital. It took Medicare 13 years to recognize the validity of outpatient surgery after the first surgicenter was built in Phoenix.

The shorthand used over and over to describe our center is "mini-hospital," which at first I found acceptable. But as time goes by, I find that description misleading. We operate a real hospital with all the services appropriate to the care of the patients we admit. In my judgment, the Fresno Recovery Care Center is no longer a pilot program. We have shown that it works, and that it is an even better idea than we had ever imagined.

MR. TONY CARR received his undergraduate education from Villanova University (B.A.), and his master of science degree in social administration from Case Western Reserve University, Cleveland, Ohio. He has been a hospital planner for the Comprehensive Health Planning Council Incorporated, Philadelphia; assistant director of the Executive Development Institute, Tulane University School of Public Health, New Orleans; and director of planning and development for Saint Mary's Medical Center, Green Bay, Wisconsin. Mr. Carr was then appointed assistant director of hospitals, Indiana University Hospitals, Indianapolis, where he also taught marketing in the Graduate School for Hospital Administration. Later he became vice-president for corporate development at Saint Agnes Medical Center, Fresno, California. He now is chief executive of the Fresno Surgery Center and Recovery Care Center. Mr. Carr serves on the boards of the California Ambulatory Surgery Association, the Northern California Ambulatory Surgery Center Association, and the Federated Ambulatory Surgery Association. He is founding president of the Indiana Society of Hospital Planning. He is active with the Rotary Club of Fresno. Mr. Carr is available as a consultant in the development of ambulatory surgery centers and recovery care centers.

12

A New Approach to Professional Liability Coverage

Marvin Rawitch, M.D.

In 1975, California physicians faced a professional liability insurance crisis. Commercial insurance carriers increased their premiums by more than 400 percent, and all the companies offering malpractice insurance were considering discontinuing the coverage. They claimed that the old premiums plus the insurers' investment income could not make up severe losses caused by skyrocketing claims and defense costs. Suddenly, a form of insurance that physicians had taken for granted for many years was threatened. The crunch quickly emerged as a major political issue.

The chaos and public controversy intensified as physicians organized mass protests and withheld medical services in limited job actions that resembled strikes. Various professional societies in California attempted to play a role in solving the crisis legislatively. Some attempted to get the ear of Governor Edmund "Jerry" Brown Jr., who worked with allies in the state Assembly to file a bill that would require all California physicians to purchase malpractice insurance from a state fund as a condition of licensure. Virtually all of the state's physicians and medical organizations opposed this proposal and called it a draconian solution.

A New Approach to Professional Liability Coverage

The special interest groups wasted no time in swapping accusations about who was most responsible for this crisis. Insurance companies blamed trial lawyers for what they called the courts' liberalization of liability doctrines in California. Trial lawyers accused the insurance companies of massive profiteering and fraud and insisted that the incidence and severity of medical negligence were on the rise. From the physicians' standpoint, it was difficult to tell what was really going on and what the various players' motives really were.

Whatever the cause of this crisis, the physicians' initial response was to form physician-owned insurance companies all over the state. Some were organized and sponsored by local medical societies. Others were set up by physician groups that structured their firms under existing state insurance laws, which set minimum capitalization requirements for fledgling companies. At the same time the medical profession and others maintained that the legal system desperately needed tort reform. To us, the courts seemed to be the prime cause of rising liability costs in California.

In 1976, the Legislature enacted the Medical Injury Compensation Reform Act (MICRA), a law that gave insurance carriers a fighting chance to provide liability insurance in California. Despite this measure, most of the commercial carriers withdrew from the market and openly encouraged physician groups to create captive funds to insure California physicians. To them, there was simply no safe way to sell malpractice insurance in the state.

This was an important factor in the very unlikely emergence of the Mutual Protection Trust of the Cooperative of American Physicians (CAP/MPT). The insurance industry lobby in Sacramento has long been the most powerful in the state, and only because it withdrew from the market and encouraged physicians to arrange their own coverage were we able to muster the political muscle to form an organization like CAP/MPT.

I became involved in December, 1975, at a medical staff meeting of a hospital in the Orange County community of Tustin. A physician and a business consultant addressed us about California's liability problems. The consultant had been retained by a small core group of Los Angeles physicians to form an entity called the Cooperative of American Physicians (CAP) that would form a self-insurance trust.

These consultants outlined a plan to have physicians join the trust by contributing refundable deposits to a fund that would generate earnings to pay for defense costs and claims against members. Each member would assume full liability, in the form of potential assessments, for expenditures beyond the funds earned by the trust.

I found the idea most intriguing because those of us who had examined conventional liability insurance realized there was no money tree that magically paid our malpractice claims. We all had gone through our professional lives under the assumption that you paid a few dollars for an insurance policy that you put away and didn't worry about. If a year went by and you didn't get sued, you lost the bet with the insurance company. If a claim was filed, you won your bet and came out ahead of the game. We labored under the mistaken notion that insurance companies had an endless supply of money available to pay claims and costs in return for our relatively meager (in former years) premiums.

Insurance companies do have a money tree of sorts. They collect premiums from policy holders, invest the money, and generate large sums that help pay claims and defense costs. But they must also pay dividends to policy holders of mutual insurance companies or dividends to stockholders of stock companies. The insurance companies also intend to collect enough premiums to pay expenses of claims asserted against those policy holders. The difference is that actuaries attempt to predict how much money will be required for each class of policy holder over an indefinite period into the future.

Prior to MICRA, the so-called "tail," or run-off period, was so open-ended and its costs so unpredictable that insurance companies believed medical liability was an uninsurable risk. Almost all of these companies for many years had absorbed underwriting losses—that is, they collected less in premiums than they were paying in claims for any group of policy holders. The difference was covered by investment income.

A New Approach to Professional Liability Coverage

In the mid-1970s, when investment income proved insufficient, insurers tried to boost premiums dramatically to make up for those losses, and this caused the crisis. With conventional liability insurance, a policy holder theoretically is paying money in advance to a company that accumulates earnings and uses the total to pay his share of claims and defense costs at some time in the future.

The idea behind the inter-indemnity trust, which was formulated by CAP, was for the trust to adopt a "pay-as-you-go" plan. We would pay a refundable premium into this trust which would generate income to cover claims and defense and administrative costs, but the money would also function as a security deposit against future assessments against the members if the trust's income were insufficient. In the event a member failed to pay an assessment, he would forfeit his deposit and lose all his protection and coverage.

I found the concept intriguing. This form of payment had to be the most efficient, I concluded, because it permitted trust members rather than the insurance companies to control the money until it was needed for claims. We could form an elite group of policy holders who would be carefully screened. Only physicians whose likelihood of generating claims would be minimal, based upon past professional performance and competence as judged by their peers, would be admitted as members. The idea sounded great to me, and the hospital staff appointed me as a committee of one to investigate.

When I contacted the group, it immediately invited me to become actively involved, and soon I joined its board of directors. But existing California law made it a violation of the insurance code for a group of physicians who were unrelated by partnership or other business arrangement to form an inter-indemnity trust. We were saddled with the burdens of not only formulating this organization, but also of approaching the California Legislature to amend the insurance code to permit such entities.

This was an uphill battle. People in the insurance business immediately claimed the idea was preposterous, unworkable, and doomed to fail even if it were permitted. The magic words were "unfunded liability," the watchwords of the insurance industry.

Assemblyman Fred Chel of Long Beach originally was approached by a group of local orthopedic surgeons to find a solution to the malpractice crisis. Chel also was sought out by CAP's founding group, five Hollywood area physicians who wanted legislation enacted to remove the legal barriers to a trust.

That bill contained the basic framework that still exists in the CAP/MPT organization, although it was primitive in that it was inflexible and did not permit a broad range of risk classes that we now take for granted. It didn't even allow for the risk classes which were then prevalent in the insurance industry. At the same time many other physician groups in California were quickly launching new traditional insurance companies because all they had to do was conform to existing regulations.

But we believed the CAP/MPT organization should be made available as an alternative to conventional insurance, and we doggedly pursued our efforts. At the time, even a new company's policies were based on unknown experience. While virtually all the professional liability insurance in California had been written on an occurrence basis (the policy covered all claims arising out of incidents occurring during the policy period, irrespective of when the claim was filed), the new companies used the so-called claims-made system (covering claims from incidents occurring during the policy period, but the claim must be reported while the insured is still a policy holder). This is more restrictive but it avoids the necessity of having to predict costs far into the future. The MICRA act was also working its way through the Legislature and was eventually adopted in 1976. Without that tort reform, it's doubtful that any insurance company or CAP/MPT could have succeeded.

We worked very hard, spending many days in Sacramento discussing these issues with assemblymen and senators. Many physicians were involved in this effort, and with the crisis atmosphere we brought the bill before the Assembly and then the Senate with overwhelming votes in our favor. The bill was introduced as urgency legislation, which required a three-quarters vote in each house. Upon passage and signature by Governor

Brown, the bill would take effect immediately instead of the following January.

Well, we achieved all that in spite of Brown's interest in having the state take over the medical liability insurance industry. When the bill finally wound up on his desk in the summer of 1976, it sat there for a long time and he didn't sign it. Many voices in his administration urged him to sign it, but the insurance commissioner, Wesley Kinder, told him not to. Kinder warned that the bill would allow organizations to operate with unfunded liability. We pointed out that the liability was actually well funded by the total net worth of all the physician members who would be responsible for assessments if necessary. Some said the physicians wouldn't join the trust for that very reason— they wouldn't permit unlimited liability to invade their net worth.

Just a few minutes before midnight on the day the bill would have become law without the governor's signature, Brown vetoed the measure. Brown might have taken this action because Kinder apparently told him he would resign if the bill were not vetoed. This type of insurance entity would open a "Pandora's Box" and permit special interest groups to leave the safe haven of the insurance industry and create self-insurance schemes that would endanger the public, he argued. In his view, only an insurance company could protect consumers from the various forms of liability.

This happened despite our group's luncheon with the governor, at which we made a contribution for his reelection campaign, to explain to him our agenda. We told him that we were simply following his political and social philosophy, which recognized that we lived in an era of limits. Government could not do everything, and citizens had to do more for themselves. We agreed with him and told him we did not believe government should take over the control and issuance of professional medical liability insurance as he proposed. Instead, physicians should do it themselves through the formation of physician-owned malpractice insurance carriers and the alternative we proposed, which we felt would provide coverage at less cost. Our underwriting would be more stringent, and the physicians' knowledge that their pocketbooks would be subject to unlimited assessments would modify their behavior. We would be careful in choosing physician members so we could operate at lower cost. Governor Brown didn't have much to say, although he seemed to listen. He wound up vetoing the bill anyway.

Naturally we were devastated. We had all worked very hard and spent a great deal of personal time and money on this, and our dreams were dashed. A member of the Assembly Finance, Insurance and Commerce Committee, the key committee in process, came to the rescue. Tom Bain was a knowledgeable senior Assemblyman. Because this was the second session of the Legislature, we could not introduce a new bill, so Bain suggested we find another live bill that had a committee hearing, take it over as our own and make another run at the Legislature.

Finance, Insurance and Commerce Committee member Richard Robinson, a freshman assemblyman, said he had such a bill that was not important to him or his constituents and offered it to us. We "hijacked" the bill, amended our language into it, changed the title and made changes in the law in response to the governor's veto message. In three weeks we had brought the bill through the Assembly and the Senate again. The votes were overwhelmingly in our favor—far greater than the three-quarters needed for the urgency legislation that helped us avoid waiting until the next year for the law to take effect.

Once again, the bill wound up on the governor's desk. Once again it sat there, and Brown did nothing. Intensive lobbying continued. The insurance commissioner argued against the bill. Insurance industry interests lobbied against it (secretly, we believed), and even some of the newly formed doctor-owned insurance companies joined them.

The California Medical Association counseled us about lobbying and recommended that the trust concept be offered as an alternative. The medical association did not take a position that this was superior to conventional insurance, but the organization and its president, Kash Rose, M.D., and its legislative assistant, Jay Michaels, gave us encouragement for which we will always be grateful.

We were coming down to the wire again. Many others had urged the governor not to veto the bill because it dealt with the malpractice crisis, a very hot topic in the public's mind, and that if the crazy doctors wanted to do this unconventional thing, he should allow them to do it even if he thought it might not be the best thing. Again he worried about unfunded liability, and we kept pointing out that it was really not unfunded. It was funded by the deep pockets of every physician member. In many ways, we argued, it was an even stronger financial base than the insurance companies had because they merely had to meet minimum capital requirements. If we were to add the total assets of all the MPT participants, they would far exceed the insurance company capitalization and reserve requirements.

The governor still wouldn't sign the bill, but he didn't veto it either. In the early fall of 1976, it became law without his signature—30 days after its enactment.

At last, we had the law. Now we had to persuade enough qualified physicians to join the organization. The trust needed at least 500 doctors with an average contribution of $20,000 each to reach the $10-million minimum.

We had to live with restrictions on how we could share the risk. Conventional insurance companies had always been able to assign different medical specialties different degrees of risk. Among the nine risk classifications, policy holders paid a wide range of premiums for the same coverage. But our contribution and assessment range was very narrow, from $17,500 to $22,500. Members of low-risk specialties, such as general practitioners, dermatologists, allergists, and radiologists, correctly saw this as unfair because high-risk neurosurgeons, orthopedists, and obstetricians had to pay only slightly more. I was disappointed that we had to do that, but I believed then it still would be better than conventional insurance. I also was convinced that as the organization matured and grew, this restriction would be brought into line with other carriers.

I spent many hours traveling around the state, addressing medical staff meetings, physician groups, and individuals to explain the trust, its philosophy, and how it would work in the best interests of its members. By early 1977 we finally signed up the necessary physicians and collected $10 million in provisional contributions. We officially opened for business.

It was learn as you go. We made some mistakes early on. The majority of the original boards of directors and trustees believed the cooperative organization should offer other services to physicians, ranging from car leasing to a credit union. I thought that was a mistake, that the organization should concentrate only on offering low-cost liability insurance. But my viewpoint did not prevail, and the organization began to expand its scope.

In 1979, after about 18 months of operation, there was a very open split in the organization. The dissident faction questioned the way things were done and whether the organization should provide anything other than liability insurance. A special meeting was called and all the directors and trustees resigned. The company reorganized with a brand new board of directors of CAP and a brand new board of trustees of MPT, and it's all been getting better since then.

We didn't have our first assessment until 1984. Our current costs are much lower than those of any other carrier in California, and we have lowered "premiums" and refunded assessments three years in a row. Many of the concepts we originated were adopted by other carriers. We initiated "nose," or retroactive, coverage, which other insurers now commonly offer. We pioneered a plan allowing a physician to remain covered after reaching retirement age without making further payments regardless of claims made. Other carriers required those doctors to continue paying regular premiums at the time of the occurrence and when the claim was reported. We also initiated the idea of suspending assessments for physicians during periods of disability. CAP/MPT currently provides coverage to more than 3,500 California physicians and is growing at 9 percent per year.

MICRA has succeeded in reducing liability costs, and instead of being the premium cost leader, California now is doing relatively well compared with other states that have failed to pass significant tort reform. All the major provisions of MICRA have been upheld by the California Supreme Court, and our organization faces as bright a future as is possible in today's rough and tumble political, social, and economic climate.

A New Approach to Professional Liability Coverage

MARVIN RAWITCH, M.D., received his undergraduate education at Northwestern University, Evanston, Illinois, and his medical education at the Medical School, University of Illinois, Chicago. Following a rotating internship at the Illinois Masonic Hospital, Chicago, he served his residency in radiology at the Illinois Masonic Hospital and Los Angeles County General Hospital. Dr. Rawitch fulfilled his military obligations as a captain in the U.S. Army Reserves. He is a Diplomate of the American Board of Radiology in Diagnosis, Therapy, and Nuclear Medicine, and a Fellow of the American College of Radiology. He is a founding director and trustee of the Mutual Protection Trust of the Cooperative of American Physicians, and past president and director of the Foothill Communities Association, Santa Ana, California. He is in the private practice of radiology in Orange County, California. Dr. Rawitch is available as a consultant in the field of inter-indemnity trust development for professional liability coverage.

13

Preferred and Exclusive Provider Groups

Harvey E. Knoernschild, M.D., M.Med.Sci.

Preferred provider contracting is the fastest growing health care delivery system in the United States today. Since 1982, preferred provider organizations (PPOs) have been offered as an alternative system to the traditional indemnity insurance plans and to health maintenance organizations (HMOs). During the early 1990s more than 50 percent of the insured population will be covered by a PPO-based health care plan, according to projections; 35 percent will be HMO members; and only 15 percent will continue to receive coverage in the indemnity system. With premiums increasing 25 to 60 percent a year, employers and other payers understandably have become pessimistic about traditional health care funding. They want alternatives. Facing the specter of mandatory health insurance for their employees at unaffordable rates, many businesses claim they will be threatened if health care costs are not stabilized. National health insurance, often discussed and openly scorned by organized medicine, is attracting more interest and support from business, labor, government, and even the medical community itself.

Because of these pressures, many believe that the PPO health care delivery system is the final bastion of "fee-for-service" medical practice in America. Physicians are being warned that unless they can work effectively and efficiently within PPO guidelines, they will soon be salaried by a government agency or an HMO. Certainly, new approaches to health care delivery must be implemented soon in every community if the traditional American fee-for-service system is to survive seven more years. Recognition of this has led to the new generation of smaller preferred provider groups known as exclusive provider organizations (EPOs).

One such EPO, the "risk-EPO," is a hybrid of the PPO and HMO prototypes which blends the discounted fee-for-service features of a PPO with the physician risk-sharing aspects of an HMO. The risk-EPO is a significant move toward "managed health care." Its success depends on an innovative financing structure, improved preventive medical practice habits, an enlightened dedication to cost-efficiency, and creative benefit design. Managed health care is the future, but the basic issues are quality and cost. According to a recent report by InterStudy, the Minneapolis health care think tank, "The winners in the 1990s and beyond will be those health care plans that can document delivery of high quality care in an efficient manner."

Many physicians are unaware of how a PPO/EPO group can benefit their own practices. The actual formation of a PPO/EPO is not difficult or complex, assuming that it is done by a group of dedicated and informed physicians who comprehend the trends in health care delivery and want to occupy the best competitive position. It requires adequate background information, a dedicated core leadership group, a membership willing to police itself, a commitment to efficient practice, and enlightened payers and employers who want to reduce their costs. Of course, there will be some risk-taking, and the faint of heart may not want to participate initially. But as the PPO/EPO group builds its patient/ client base and efficiently provides quality care, membership will become very attractive.

In this chapter, we will review the evolutionary development, classification, advantages, and deficiencies of preferred provider groups, as well as how a group of physicians can develop its own PPO/EPO. Of course, the author is not an attorney, and all information and opinions are based on his personal experience in the development of three PPO/EPOs. Anyone attempting this project should obtain competent legal assistance.

EVOLUTION OF PREFERRED PROVIDER ORGANIZATIONS

Health care costs have escalated rapidly during the past 15 years. Most recently, medical costs have increased 25 to 80 percent a year for employers. In many industries, health care expenses are among the most significant costs of doing business. In fact, Chrysler Corporation Chairman Lee Iacocca stated that in 1978 his company spent more on health insurance premiums than it did on steel or tires. From coast to coast, corporate executives pursued new solutions. Employers have come to believe that cost and employee satisfaction are the top priorities in health care benefit plans. Indemnity plans had grown too expensive, but HMOs were not always accepted by employees. By reviewing these two "extremes," we can follow the development of the PPO system and its inevitable hybrid, the exclusive provider group.

In the insurance world, a PPO refers to the combined network of physician groups and hospitals providing health care services under discounted contracts. For our purposes, a PPO is a group of professional providers, such as physicians, dentists, chiropractors, etc., who have banded together to contract with employers or payers to provide services at discounted fees in exchange for an increased volume of patients. Usually the PPO is linked with one or more hospitals that offer a per diem rate or other contract discount. The PPO is usually set up as a corporation, with each provider member being an equal stockholder. The relationship of each individual provider to the others is loose and non-binding. PPO expenses for administrative and secretarial support, legal fees, etc., are paid via annual dues. The board of directors is elected by the membership, which in turn elects officers and appoints committees.

An EPO is generally a PPO with fewer members who become the exclusive providers for a payer with a specific client base. The patient has fewer hospital and facility selections in the EPO system. Physician fee discounts may be greater in an EPO. The legal structure is generally the same, although it is common for the affiliation to be more tightly structured, such as with a clinic or an independent practice association. Recently, a variant of the EPO has emerged—a risk-EPO, which offers a PPO-type contract with a 10 to 20 percent "withhold" on physician fees. The withhold is not paid to the providers at the end of the fiscal year if they have overspent the allocated budget for services rendered. If the EPO group has been successful in meeting or exceeding budget targets, the withhold is paid. Members of the EPO may also share surplus funds left in the budget at year end. The risk-EPO contains some unique features for improving cost controls and is a blend of the PPO and HMO. From this point on, EPO will refer to the "risk-type" EPO model.

BASIC HEALTH CARE SYSTEMS

Indemnity Plans: Total access with no cost-control. Traditional insurance plans have quite obviously become too expensive. To believe that this form of health care financing will return is like waiting for the dinosaurs to re-emerge and flourish on the face of the earth. However, we should salvage the good features and incorporate them into new alternatives.

Employee satisfaction has always been highest with the indemnity system of health care delivery because of its virtually unlimited access. An employee or family member could see virtually any physician or hospital with confidence that they would receive medical care. However, there were no restrictions on the number of tests or days in the hospital. In the "good old days" up to the 1970s, physicians didn't worry about utilization review, cost containment, pre-admission certification, or any of the features existing now with managed health care. Physicians were paid their usual, customary, and reasonable (UCR) fees, without considering the prospect of a claims audit or review. Preserving a large physician access pool becomes a most desirable feature in the eyes of the patient, and limitations become quite conspicuous.

As new technologies came along, physicians justified acquisition of expensive diagnostic and therapeutic marvels with the classic rationale: "I want whatever is best for my patients." But all too often, the new technology was put into use by physicians who didn't fully understand its appropriate role in their practices. Little or no information was given to the ordering physician about indications and contraindications for the test or study. Hospitals were pressured into purchasing the latest equipment by their medical staffs or by competition with a neighboring hospital that had purchased it, or both. To justify the purchase, the hospital administration presented financial projections showing the equipment would "pay for itself" in 12 or 18 months. No one cared what the charges were going to be. The patient bought the insurance policy and the insurance company extracted its expenses and profit and paid the bills. Any shortage was recovered the next year when the premium was increased. Those were the so-called "golden years" of American medicine because everyone got what they wanted. Many believe that this blindness to cost trends by insurance companies was a major factor in precipitating the current health care crisis.

Yet there are lessons to be learned from the traditional indemnity plans, and we must apply them in the future. Most patients want to choose their providers from a large number of physicians and hospitals. They don't like to be restricted. They also want every conceivable test and study which they read about in popular magazines to be available to them on demand. They believe that high quality care is synonymous with expensive care. The challenge for the employer who pays for the care and for the physician who provides it is to educate and convince the patient that high-quality health care doesn't require every test or study available to arrive at a diagnosis, nor does it require access to every physician or hospital. A preferred or exclusive provider group is a first step in reducing the number of physicians and facilities available to the patient in exchange for a smaller health care bill. But this program imposes a responsibility on the PPO/EPO to select and keep only those physicians who provide quality and cost-effective care. Members who use excessive tests or studies, obtain unnecessary consultations, or perform unnecessary surgery must be reeducated or removed. The economic survival of the group takes precedence over any individual member. This is basic to a successful PPO/EPO.

Health Maintenance Organizations: Restricted access but tough cost controls. The prepaid medical program originated in 1929 when two physicians established a plan for Los Angeles Department of Water and Power employees and their families. Four years later, on the Mojave Desert in Southern California, Dr. Sidney Garfield started caring for construction workers at a daily "capitated" rate of 5 cents per worker regardless of how much care he gave to any individual worker. In 1937, Henry J. Kaiser asked Dr. Garfield to set up a similar program for workers building the Grand Coulee Dam in Washington state. The Kaiser-Permanente Plan, the largest and most successful prepaid medical coverage plan, emerged from the construction industry. The term "health maintenance organization" was coined by Dr. Paul Ellwood, Jr., a Minneapolis physician and longtime proponent of prepaid care.

Although HMOs have existed since the 1930s, many patients then and now have found HMOs too restrictive in provider and hospital selection. They complained of long waits to get appointments and then long waits in physician waiting rooms. Often patients were unable to have their "own doctor" and would be seen instead by the first available clinic physician. This prompted many HMO patients to see a community physician outside the HMO plan and pay the fee out of their own pockets.

Without question, the early HMOs achieved remarkable cost control, but this apparently occurred at the expense of quality. The working philosophy of these plans apparently was to delay or avoid treating beneficiaries who suffered from non-life threatening conditions. Because the HMO providers shared in the plan profits (the residual funds in the "capitation pool" at the end of the year, for example), many outsiders believed that the HMO physician's judgment was inappropriately motivated by the financial reward for doing less. Any savings in the budget at the end of the year went to the physician-partner as a bonus, or incentive reward. For many years, this system led to concerns regarding the quality and quantity of medical care delivered by

HMOs. Physicians who worked for HMOs often were slighted by their peers and local medical associations.

Times have changed, and public perceptions of the quality of care rendered by large HMOs have improved over the past several years. Through improved selection of physicians and smart public relations and advertising, HMOs are having considerable success shedding the old image. With the current HMO market share at about 35 percent nationwide and about 65 percent of the labor force in some areas, it is the fastest growing health care option. To counter the perception that HMOs ration services to produce a profit, some are now starting to look for areas of "underservice" and to evaluate the competency of their physician gatekeepers. In general, the prepaid, capitated HMO system of health insurance will be around for a long time, and PPO/EPOs must study their cost-efficiency methods.

Several lessons can be learned from the HMO system before PPO/EPOs can even try to compete with them. Foremost among these is that the physician must bear a financial risk to make the delivery system efficient. Whether this is achieved by means of a withhold or a bonus, the provider must have a monetary incentive to meet predetermined targets or expense levels. Fee-for-service practices can still be maintained, but a reward for efficiency is a practical and necessary way to achieve compliance with utilization goals. There must be a physician-directed prospective utilization review service managing the use of expensive studies, procedures, and hospital admissions. Data collection that allows the PPO/EPO to accurately evaluate the performance of each member must be incorporated into the review. This review service must be responsive to the medical necessity and appropriateness of the attending physician's request, as well as to the cost-effective alternatives available within the local community. For these reasons, the reviewers must be respected, high-quality physicians from within the group itself. Each reviewer must have a passion for efficiency and encourage his or her peers to do the same. If the forming PPO/EPO is unable to do this task internally, outside companies can tailor a review program to fit the needs of the PPO/EPO.

TYPES OF PREFERRED PROVIDER ORGANIZATIONS

There are three major types of PPOs, with the classification based on the sponsoring agency or group that forms the PPO. The following criteria can be used to compare each type:

- Quality control of physician membership selection.
- Disciplinary actions available for use against members.
- Internal monitoring of members' cost-efficiency habits.
- Ability and desire of the PPO to modify practice habits.

Provider-sponsored PPOs. Most hospitals have encouraged the formation of medical staff PPOs in order to enter the growing PPO market. Hospitals began networking with other hospitals to provide wide geographical coverage, such as SelectHEALTH in California. Some of these networks merged into larger organizations with even greater coverage, such as SelectHEALTH into Preferred Health Network.

The quality of physicians in this type of PPO can vary considerably and is generally dependent on the criteria for medical staff membership, the PPO selection process, and internal disciplinary activities. With some groups, all physicians with admitting privileges at the hospital are eligible to join. Others carefully examine utilization data from the hospital to select physicians who use hospital resources efficiently. Evaluating a provider's outpatient efficiency is nearly impossible without input from the insurance company or third-party administrator. Few PPOs have terminated members for inefficiency, but they have done so for loss or restriction of hospital privileges. In general, the physicians in this group of PPOs have the potential for being of the highest quality, because peers within the hospital setting know who the high-quality practitioners are.

The utilization review imposed on provider-sponsored PPOs is the choice of the individual payer. Long-distance review is the most common, but the data obtained by the review are not shared with the group, and internal monitoring is thereby prevented. Few companies will delegate review to the PPO itself, fearing that "the fox would be watching the hen house" and inappropriate services would not be controlled. However, this is changing as the PPO model evolves into an EPO model. Hospitals are capable of keeping basic utilization data on the members of their own medical staffs and can provide the data to their affiliated PPO/EPO.

Payer-sponsored PPOs (insurance companies). As soon as insurance companies discovered that physicians were willing to discount fees to maintain patient base, they developed their own PPOs. Most carriers have replaced their indemnity plans with PPO-options designed to lower premiums through discounted contract fees with physicians and facilities. In many instances, all physicians receiving fee-for-service payments from insurers received an application to join their PPO. Those who returned an application in a timely manner were included in the insurance company's PPO roster. No further quality controls of any significance were applied.

Insurance companies have amassed considerable billing and other data that are vital to cost-containment. Unfortunately, little of this data has been shared with the providers generating the expenses or with the PPO that could use it to counsel a member and attempt to change inefficient practice habits. Undoubtedly, this data eventually will be used to cull out providers who fail to meet utilization standards. Payer-sponsored PPOs usually conduct their own utilization reviews or contract them out to a proprietary review company. Again, the PPO is not given the responsibility for doing its own utilization review. As EPOs emerge, utilization management finally is being passed to the physician group, partly because the insurance industry recognized that its review system has been ineffective in controlling health care costs.

Commercial PPOs ("mail-order" PPOs). With the rapid expansion of the PPO marketplace, medical and non-medical entrepreneurs have developed PPOs, some extending into many states. The commercial PPOs were formed by mailing contracts to most physicians within the target area. When an adequate number and distribution of providers were under contract, the panel was marketed to payers. With a long list of potential clients available and waiting, these commercial PPOs signed up many providers at deeply discounted rates. Fee schedules with discounts of 20 to 25 percent were offered—many with restrictive and onerous terms.

The membership selection process of the commercial PPOs was weak, and few applicants were turned down. Apparently the quality of care was not as important to these groups as the rapid formation of their networks. As a result of the deep discounting and weak selection process, enrolled providers tended to be those who were less busy and perhaps of lesser quality in the community. Utilization review was conducted long-distance by review nurses and clerks with little or no effort to perform peer-to-peer utilization monitoring. Several of these PPOs do provide their members with useful cost-containment information, but they are the exception.

DIRECT PPO/EPO CONTRACTING

As employers who "weren't going to take it any more" started searching for alternatives to their existing health care system, some contracted directly with PPO physician groups and hospitals. In 1983, the Hewlett-Packard PPO was formed with physicians from El Camino Hospital in Mountain View, California, a tax-supported district hospital with an enlightened medical staff and progressive administration. This has become the model for direct contracting by a major industry.

Shortly after the Hewlett-Packard PPO was formed, the American Electronics Association (AEA) began to explore this new medical care system. Members of the AEA, including some of the largest electronics companies in Silicon Valley, began pooling their claims and utilization data. After several years and many thousands of entries into the AEA database, a plan was developed for entering into direct contractual relationships with the PPOs at several hospitals in Santa Clara County. Representatives of the human resource departments of five of the AEA companies met individually with the contract directors of the hospitals and negotiated a basic per diem rate for their employees. The hospitals learned that if they offered lower rates, the companies were willing to limit the number of contracting hospitals. The promise of a higher volume of patients to the hospital was instrumental in achieving a lower per diem rate.

After the contracts with the hospital were completed, the affiliated PPO physician groups were approached, first as a group and then individually. Although each medical staff had already formed an organization in order to respond to increasing numbers of insurance companies requesting contracts, this was our first exposure to contracting directly with the employer/payer sector. The Silicon Valley companies wanted a complete range of specialists and primary care physicians, and they offered a fee schedule which was close to the community's usual, customary, and reasonable fee profile. With counsel from an attorney specializing in health care, the contract was negotiated point by point, and after several months, the final PPO-physician agreement was reached.

The physician contracts were mailed to each PPO member, and after many phone calls and discussions, the majority of members signed and returned the contract. We met the deadline the companies imposed so they could print materials and rosters for the employee sign-up campaign.

Direct contracting with employers forges a close and dynamic relationship between industry and medicine. Physicians learn to appreciate the impact health care costs have on a company and are stimulated to improve their own efficiency. The employer is encouraged by the medical group to add wellness programs and other preventive medical benefits to the employee plan. Each can learn from the other how to improve the quality of care for the employee/patient.

THE FAILURE OF TRADITIONAL PPOs

When physician-fee discounting first became prevalent, there was a great expectation that this would rapidly reduce health care costs. But after seven years, this has not occurred—at least not to the extent first predicted. Simply paying a physician or hospital less for a provided service has not reversed the inflationary elements in medicine, and it cannot be expected to. There are many reasons for this.

Ineffective utilization review. Most utilization review today is conducted by long-distance telephone by nurses, clerks, or retired physicians. Very seldom does a peer physician in active practice in the same community discuss management of a case with the attending physician. This is a shortsighted policy, because it has little long-term impact on altering the habits of the inefficient and wasteful attending physician. If, on the other hand, respected, high-quality, and cost-conscious local physicians would become actively involved, utilization review could have a significant impact on poor practice routines.

Inadequate education on proper uses of new technology. The most rapidly growing health care costs are those generated by outpatient services. Often new technology used in the outpatient environment has already advanced to clinical trial status before its appropriate role in clinical medicine is fully determined. Physicians who order these new studies without fully understanding the indications for appropriate use are wasting resources if a simpler and less expensive test produces the same result. In many cases, tests are ordered which will not be used in determining the diagnosis or in changing the way a patient is treated.

Discounted fee schedules may cause abuse. Discounting does not always produce lower health care costs, and it may actually increase overall costs. Many physicians have no need to discount their fees or to join PPOs because the quality of their services are recognized by their peers and their practices are already sufficiently busy.

Within any community, there will always be a small number of providers who, because of greed, avarice, or declining income, resort to unethical business practices to increase their incomes. For them, discounting may produce an incentive to resort to abusive methods in order to recoup their revenue. Here are some of the more common abuses that insurance companies have observed:

"Creative pricing" tricks are the most frequently used abuses. "Code-creep" is one example in which a provider submits a fee to the insurance company for doing more than was actually done. For example, a mole measuring 2 mm in diameter is removed, but it becomes 10 mm in size on the insurance claim.

"Unbundling services" is a technique in which the surgeon separates each step of an operation into its components. A cholecystectomy conceivably could be billed as (1) an exploratory laparotomy (the abdomen is opened), (2) exploration of the retroperitoneum (the common duct is exposed), (3) exploration of the common duct (a small probe is passed through the cystic duct into the common duct), (4) lysis of adhesions (small adhesive bands are divided), and finally (5) cholecystectomy (the gallbladder is removed). Although unbundling is done routinely in some paramedical fields, it is not to be tolerated and should not be accepted by insurance companies.

"Yo-yoing" is self-referral. Sometimes a provider who owns an expensive piece of equipment is tempted to exaggerate the indications and overuse the instrument within his or her office practice. What goes on inside the physician's office is seldom known to the outside world. The indications for performing a test can be stretched quite easily. It is more difficult for this to occur in settings where there are built-in "peerwatch" mechanisms, such as hospital medical care evaluation committees that review medical records, and anesthesiologists and pathologists who watch surgeons.

"Ping-ponging" is creating unnecessary referrals to associates who reciprocate. The patient becomes the ball and is bounced back and forth from provider to provider to extract fees from insurers for inappropriate services. Sometimes the mere hint of a symptom by a patient is used as an opportunity to play ping-pong.

Although probably less than 5 percent of providers actually engage in fee padding, it has been estimated that this accounts for up to 25 percent of all health care costs. Most of these unscrupulous physicians are known to their peers in the medical community. Identifying these providers and excluding them from managed health care contracts is essential if health care costs are to be reduced and the PPO/EPO is to stay in business.

Providers are not at risk in a PPO contract. With the exception of risking the non-renewal of a contract, physicians and other providers are not at risk in the current PPO contract system. Payers are aware of this and point to this deficiency as one reason why the PPO-experiment has not produced the anticipated savings. Risk-EPOs, which are midway between HMOs and PPOs, are already coming into the marketplace. Risk-EPO proponents contend physicians will behave in a more cost-conscious manner if they are placed at risk through the withholding of a portion of their fees. There is good logic in this approach, and the first EPOs are being carefully watched by the insurance industry. If successful, it is likely that most insurance carriers will follow suit. A PPO in the formation stages must educate its members about the inevitability of risk-EPO contracting.

Lack of patient self-responsibility. Patients must be motivated by their physicians and health plans to take more responsibility for their own health care. By eliminating poor health habits, using resources carefully, and using alternative and cost-effective facilities, patients can have a significant impact on the overall cost of health care. Smoking cessation alone eventually can eliminate 30 to 35 percent of the cost of health care services. Benefit plan designs must encourage self-responsibility through company-sponsored wellness programs and effective workplace education. Increasing the financial responsibility of the patient with higher copayments and deductions is an effort in this direction. A positive incentive program must be developed, otherwise this move will be fought vigorously by unions and other organized employee groups.

EXCLUSIVE PROVIDER ORGANIZATIONS (EPOs)

Clearly, a PPO system in which the provider is not at any financial risk misses the cost-control features of an HMO. One of the perceived reasons why HMOs have been extremely successful in keeping costs and premiums down is the incentive bonus program. The physician-partner receives a portion of the savings achieved at year end. Prepaid funds not spent during the year are divided among the efficient providers. Just as the HMO group is at risk for cost overruns and excessive utilization, so does it benefit when savings are realized. This concept is being merged with PPO programs, and the risk-EPO has been introduced as a compromise between PPOs and HMOs.

In an EPO, the insurance company or self-insured employer establishes a budget goal that is experience-rated. That means the annual premium is set by an actuarially determined amount based on what it cost to pay for the medical expenses of that beneficiary group during the previous year. An inflationary "fudge factor" is added, and that becomes the budget goal for that employee group. Physicians who participate in the EPO agree to accept a withhold of 10 to 20 percent from their contracted fee schedule. The withhold accumulates in an escrow account. At the end of the contract year, if the budget goal has been achieved, the physicians receive full return of their withhold plus a portion of the residual funds in the budget. This quite neatly has placed physicians at risk for the amount of their withhold and rewarded them with an opportunity to receive a bonus if resources are conserved to a greater degree. The same physicians who are ordering the tests, the admissions, and the procedures and causing all medical health care expenses will now directly benefit for being more efficient themselves and encouraging their peers within their own group to do likewise. The concept works for HMOs, and it will work for the properly designed and developed PPO/EPO group.

The first of the risk-EPOs has been marketed, and more will follow. This model stresses the need for newly formed PPO groups to incorporate the required terms and conditions for their members, both new and continuing. All members must be team players who agree to work together to achieve the common objective. Cost-efficiency must be stressed, but without sacrificing quality. Those surgeons with excessive complication rates and longer hospitalizations will be prevented from joining the group. Cardiologists who do echocardiograms and angiograms without clear indications will be dipping into the "common pot" and placing all members at risk for the loss of their withhold funds. Such actions will not be tolerated for long.

Under the risk-EPO plan, the group itself is encouraged to do its own utilization review and monitoring. The sponsoring agents are able to continue doing the review themselves but they usually are anxious to delegate review to the PPO/EPO group. With physicians jointly at risk for excessive costs, PPO/EPOs must have or develop the personnel to conduct internal utilization management and data collection. A strong review committee must be created with every specialty represented. The payer must agree to share concurrent claims data with the group, and the group should be prepared to do its own centralized billing and data capture. The PPO/EPO must also employ the expertise to analyze the risk of any contract it enters into with a client. The services of an experienced actuary may be needed.

In summary, the risk-EPO can only function smoothly and effectively if its administration is capable of utilization review and case management, medical group development, credentialing and quality assurance, and effective promotion of cost-efficient practice habits. In my opinion, the majority of PPO contracts will convert to risk-EPO contracts by the mid-1990s.

FORMING A PPO/EPO IN YOUR COMMUNITY

Certainly the trend in the United States health care market is toward groups of providers contracting together. By the mid-1990s, only 5 to 10 per cent of patients will carry indemnity-type insurance, 50 to 60 percent will be with HMOs, and the remaining 30 to 45 percent will join a PPO/EPO managed care system. An isolated, non-contracting physician will have a hard time surviving in an urban or suburban community if this trend holds true.

Thus the prudent physician will want to participate in the contracting strength available to a larger organization. The options are to join a health maintenance organization, enter a multi-specialty clinic that contracts with both HMOs and PPO/EPOs, or remain relatively independent and join a PPO/EPO group that has the foresight to prepare for risk-taking contracts.

For those who cherish independence, we will review the process of "How to start your own PPO/EPO," or "If you can't lick 'em, join 'em."

1. Identify the key leadership group and arrange an organizational meeting. Within each medical community there are a few leaders who influence the decisions of others. Hopefully, these individuals are well known to you, but it may take some exploring and research to uncover the most appropriate leaders. If your hospital management is interested, and there is no reason it wouldn't be, ask the administrators to recommend several leaders. Perhaps they can provide you with the admissions activity of the medical staff. The medical staff secretary is a good resource for identifying unsung leaders. This core group should have at least one representative from each of the major specialties. Those in medical staff leadership may be worth including, especially if the PPO/EPO is to be based at one hospital. Invite the leadership group to an informational meeting to discuss the formation of a "contracting group."

Give at least three weeks notice of an informational and/or organizational meeting. Ten days before the meeting (any sooner and it will be misplaced), send each invitee an informational package with material on health care economics, trends, and alternative delivery systems. Use diagrams and graphics to define the features of a PPO, an EPO, an HMO, etc. Develop an organizational plan to serve as a discussion starting point. Don't call in any lawyers yet. If you want to include the hospital, ask the most respected hospital administration representative to attend and participate. Allow three hours for this first meeting, and bring extra informational packages.

Here is a suggested agenda for the meeting:

> Introductions.
> Declare purpose and goals of meeting.
> Review and discuss health care trends.
> Define terminology.
> Present an organizational plan.
> Charter a board of directors.
> Identify chairmanships to be filled by participants:
>> Membership and Quality Assurance (Priority 1).
>> Utilization Review (Priority 1).
>> Finance (Priority 1).
>> Contract Review (Priority 2).
>> Membership Services (Priority 3).
>> Public Relations (Priority 3).
> Elect a charter board of directors.

Set a meeting schedule, with sessions at least every two weeks.

2. Charter a board of directors and officers. You have to start somewhere. If the concept of forming a PPO/EPO group is acceptable to a meaningful number of those at the exploratory meeting, select a charter board of directors to make organizing decisions. The charter board could be automatically disbanded after this initial phase, although most members should remain as the first board of directors. By having this option, any member who does not perform can easily be replaced. Having a committed and actively involved board is critical to the success of any organization, including PPO/EPOs.

At the first meeting of the charter board, officers should be selected, and key committee assignments made. The board's initial tasks include selecting an attorney to explain the options available, organize the corporation, and prepare the bylaws; choosing an administrative secretary; and preparing a preliminary budget for the first year of operations, including funding sources such as sale of stock, dues, or assessments. The board must also take into account various expenses that must be budgeted, including salary and benefits for the administrative secretary; office equipment, such as computers, software, printers, telephones, an answering machine and a copier; office furniture; rent; insurance premiums for directors and officers coverage, a premises liability policy, and a workers compensation plan; supplies, printing, mailing, and miscellaneous expenses; legal fees; and a strategic planning consultant (optional).

3. Select an attorney, incorporate, and adopt a budget. After the charter board has been elected, you are ready to complete the organizational phase by choosing the best vehicle for incorporation within your state and adopting corporate bylaws and other documents—all of which requires the services of an attorney. The job can be delegated to an attorney selection subcommittee, which should interview several lawyers before making a choice. The developing PPO/EPO should find a lawyer with previous experience in health care organization to avoid paying for the education of an attorney in this specialty. Choosing an inexperienced health care lawyer also may take longer, but it would justify a reduction in the standard legal fees.

After selecting an attorney and agreeing to an hourly or global fee arrangement, the charter board should study the advice of the lawyer and choose the corporate structure that best suits the organization. There are two primary legal structures, for-profit and non-profit. The usual PPO is organized as a non-profit corporation because it is relatively inexpensive to set up and administer, and it can be started rapidly. But that structure limits the group to PPO-contracting, making it virtually impossible to expand into for-profit areas. The PPO can command discounts on a variety of membership services from outside vendors. Membership dues are charged based on the projected annual budget.

A PPO/EPO can use an IPA structure organized as a for-profit corporation. This vehicle is more costly and time-consuming to develop, but the added advantages may make it worthwhile in the long run. Advantages include the ability to expand into for-profit membership services, such as centralized billing (which also permits data collection), phone-answering services, laboratory services, personnel pools, etc. If the PPO/EPO group anticipates a commitment to risk-type contracting, this form of corporation is the better of the two.

4. Select an administrative secretary. An administrative secretary should be hired early in the organization of the PPO/EPO. The secretary will help with paperwork and receive the best education possible by working with the board and its committees during the formative months. If properly selected and educated, the secretary will become essential to the PPO/EPO's smooth operation. It is better to pay more and secure an excellent person than to sacrifice quality to reduce salary expenses. The secretary must be the employee of the PPO/EPO and not "on loan" or paid for by the hospital, an arrangement that could present conflicts of interests down the road.

The secretary must have integrity, maturity, adaptability to the many personalities of physicians and their office staffs, experience in basic computer and office procedures, bookkeeping skill, a reputation for "self-starting" without direct supervision, and the willingness and desire to launch a new program. Knowledge of medical terminology is not important, although some legal exposure would be useful. Computer skills should include database management, word processing, and desktop publishing.

5. Develop rules and regulations. The PPO/EPO rules and regulations are a formalized list of how the organization's daily business is conducted within legal guidelines. Those guidelines are contained in the corporate bylaws, which are prepared with the lawyer's advice in accordance with state law. The rules detail duties of the committees and officers and cannot conflict with the bylaws. The rules cover qualifications and conditions for membership, the method for applicants to appeal membership decisions, quotas on specialties, duties of the committees, the purchase price of stock shares, and membership fees and assessments.

6. Establish standing committees. The board of directors should create six standing committees and appoint a chairman for each. Ideally, each chairman will sit on the board. Each is responsible for assembling committees from among the interested membership. Some committees are of higher priority, and these should be formed first, using the best available physicians. As the membership expands, the lower priority committees can start functioning.

The membership and quality assurance committee (priority 1) has the initial task of overseeing the membership selection process, which must be completely fair to all applicants and precisely follow the qualification guidelines established by the board. As applications are received, the committee should evaluate each applicant, delegate individual interviews to a committee member, review the applicant's utilization data from the hospital, and make a decision. The committee makes recommendations to the board for the acceptance or rejection of each applicant. The board makes final decisions in all membership issues.

As the PPO/EPO matures, this committee evaluates quality of care issues concerning members. Referrals are usually made to this committee by the hospital's medical care evaluation committees, but they may also come from other members who see substandard care. If your hospital has instituted a late-model quality assurance program, your committee's work will be greatly simplified. Physician members should be required to authorize transfer of hospital-acquired quality assurance data to this PPO/EPO committee. If the PPO/EPO's committee finds that the member has indeed fallen below acceptable standards, the committee may recommend that the board terminate the member for the good of the group.

The utilization review committee (Priority 1) reviews data provided by the hospital or client regarding the use of health care resources by a member or the group at large. Many hospitals will furnish to an affiliated PPO/EPO the utilization data it collects on the medical staff. In addition, the PPO/EPO should always request that any client with which it contracts will provide continuing utilization data on services provided to its beneficiaries. Insurance companies for years have been collecting data and profiles on individual physicians. Recently, self-insured companies also have been accumulating similar information. Unless this information is shared with the physician groups, it is of little use in modifying physician behavior and improving cost-effectiveness.

Because many PPO/EPO contracts are presented to the group with built-in utilization review, the utilization review committee should advocate for member physicians whenever the outside review organization rebukes a member physician or denies authorizations of that member. Likewise, if a member becomes wasteful of health care resources, it is the duty of this committee to counsel the physician and encourage efficiency. In the occasional instance when a member is unable to practice cost-effectively, and counseling has fallen on deaf ears, the committee should recommend to the board that the member be terminated from the group. Only the board should have the authority to terminate. The survival of the group takes precedence over the interests of any individual member. Due process, of course, must be followed, and the guidelines embodied in the bylaws and rules must be adhered to implicitly.

The finance committee (priority 1) may be chaired by the PPO/EPO treasurer. It must develop a first-year budget based on the best "guesstimates" of anticipated expenses. Consultation with an accountant or hospital financial officer will allow more accurate predictions. Although the administrative secretary actually will make deposits and write checks, the finance committee is ultimately responsible for the organization's funds. An accountant should be hired to review the books at least four times a year and oversee payment of federal and state income taxes. A next-year budget with dues projections is prepared before the annual membership meeting for approval by the members.

The contract review committee (priority 2) is needed when the group starts doing business with clients. When the PPO movement started, there was considerable variation in the language of the contracts, but over time the objectionable clauses have been weeded out and most contracts are similar. However, several areas remain that should be carefully examined. The experienced corporate attorney will be of great help in avoiding these pitfalls. Some PPO/EPOs refer all contracts to their attorneys. After ten or 12 contracts, the contract review committee should be able to read and identify problem areas without attorney consultation. If ever in doubt, ask the attorney to review and comment.

The membership services committee (priority 3) develops services to improve physician efficiency and decrease office overhead. To start, the committee should survey the members to determine their needs and wants. The committee then can solicit proposals from vendors and select the best services at favorable rates.

The public relations committee (priority 3) oversees communications within the PPO/EPO as well as marketing to outside clients. This involves the publication of a regular newsletter with articles on recent contracts, new members, and membership services. Brochures and other materials perhaps should be designed and printed jointly with the hospital. The committee should study all means of promoting the group to the community and use the best methods.

7. Solicit and select members. The PPO/EPO leadership must make several major decisions before making a general membership solicitation. What are the quality standards for the PPO/EPO? Philosophically, do you want to exclude the "marginal" providers from the beginning, when it is relatively easy? Or do you want to assemble a larger panel and hope for the best, knowing it is much more difficult to terminate members after the panel is operational? There is immediate pressure, of course, to obtain the largest number of physicians as soon as possible because it "looks better" and markets more easily. In the past, employers and other payers wanted huge lists of providers so every employee could find his or her own doctor included. It gave a wider selection of providers to the employee.

But larger is not always better. The group size and membership quality must be carefully balanced. Employers are learning that it is more cost-effective to have a smaller panel with higher quality physicians and other professionals. Employees are often willing to give a bit on convenient access in exchange for improved quality.

When the board is prepared to solicit members, it should send an application form and a member agreement to all candidates. The secretary should include a cover letter explaining why complete information is needed, a reminder to enclose copies of various required documents, a bill for the nonrefundable application fee, and an invoice for a share of PPO stock. The stock fee is refundable if the applicant is not accepted.

The membership committee has been organized by the board of directors and instructed in the basic qualifications required of members. It must operate within these guidelines. Actual approval of membership is made by the board of directors based on the advice of the membership committee. The application form should capture all the information the committee will need to respond to future clients, who are becoming more detailed in the information they demand before agreeing to contracts with PPO/EPO groups.

The application should at a minimum yield the following information: name, office and home addresses, phone numbers, place of birth, date of birth, state medical license number with copy attached, Drug Enforcement Administration license number with copy attached, professional society and association memberships, AMA and county medical society memberships, Internal Revenue Service identification number, Social Security number, practice type (solo, association, incorporated), names and addresses of associates, professional liability insurer and coverage limits with copy attached, field of practice and subspecialty, board certification with copy attached, medical school, internship, residencies, previous locations in practice, hospital staff memberships, percentage of practice at each hospital, disciplinary actions, restriction of privileges, and malpractice suits.

The application form should include a signed release so the PPO/EPO can obtain or verify any information to support the application. This release should grant the group the right to obtain concurrent quality assurance and utilization data from all of the physician's hospitals. Many hospitals collect basic utilization data on all staff physicians. Average length of stays (ALOS), average discharge charges, and percentage of discharges exceeding ALOS sometimes are available by diagnosis related groupings. Having this basic data on potential members is quite valuable if the PPO/EPO intends to establish a reputation as a cost-effective organization. It is doubly valuable if the PPO/EPO gets into risk-EPO or HMO contracting, because the efficiency of a single member can affect the income of the entire membership. Patient confidentiality must be protected, but the group must have the right to view this information to assure employers that beneficiaries are receiving the highest quality and most cost-efficient care possible. The application can also include an agreement to submit disputes with the PPO/EPO to binding arbitration.

A nonrefundable application fee should be charged to cover the cost of processing and verifying information. Only after the physician has returned the completed application with a signed member agreement, the fee, and a check for the stock should the secretary submit the package to the membership committee. All funds should be deposited in an interest-bearing account. If the applicant is not accepted, the accumulated interest should be refunded with the original stock purchase charge.

The membership committee should screen applications in accordance with the expressed philosophy of the board of directors. It is essential that the membership guidelines be applied evenly to each applicant. If the committee needs additional information to make a decision, the applicant should be notified of a delay. Each applicant should be interviewed by a member of the membership committee. This allows for an exchange of information about the PPO/EPO and indicates to the applicant that membership is taken seriously. The committee member reports impressions of the applicant at the next committee meeting.

Minutes of the membership committee should be retained, with each decision recorded as accepted, deferred (usually while awaiting further information), or not accepted. A holding category may be useful to indicate that a quota is full and that the applicant will be accepted when space opens. Payment for stock is kept for the accepted applications, returned for the not accepted and holding applicants, and held until a final decision is made for the deferred group. The board of directors makes final membership decisions because it usually is the only entity protected by the PPO/EPO's liability insurance policy for directors and officers. Committee members may not be covered.

There are practical reasons why the PPO/EPO may want to limit the number of physicians in each field of practice. First, a physician's office staff is often working with contracts that have different requirements for pre-admission or pre-testing certification, copayments, billings, etc. They need to handle a minimum volume of PPO/EPO patients to become proficient in following these guidelines. If the staff sees only a rare patient from a given contract, paperwork is more likely to be managed inaccurately. This may subject the patient and physician to unneeded financial burdens. Second, the physician who practices efficiently is able to reduce the cost of health care for that given patient and is working to continue the contract when PPO/EPO renewal time comes. Thus it is in the best interest of the group to limit membership to the best and most efficient providers. Only as the volume of patients increases to a significant level should the group place additional physicians on the roster. The definition of "significant level" is open to debate, but existing groups have used a quota that produces a 20-percent practice penetration.

The following distribution of physicians produces an approximate 20-percent practice penetration for 20,000 covered employees and dependents:

Anesthesiology	7
Family/general practice	33
General surgery	10
Internal medicine and subspecialties	25
Obstetrics/gynecology	20
Ophthalmology	5
Orthopedic surgery including hand	5
Pathology	3
Pediatrics	10
Psychiatry	10
Radiology	7
Urology	4
Cardiac surgery	3
Vascular surgery	3
Thoracic surgery	3
Plastic surgery	2
Total	150

This is a rough guideline. More or fewer physicians in any specialty may be needed based on the demographics of the beneficiary population. But when scaled to size, this offers a convenient starting point.

The membership agreement spells out the terms of the understanding between the PPO/EPO and the member. The member and the PPO/EPO each agree to certain considerations:

1. The physician allows the PPO/EPO to market the PPO/EPO, to represent the member in contract negotiations, and to forward all offers to the member.

2. The member can choose not to participate in any contract.

3. The member pledges to provide cost-effective, high-quality medical care to beneficiaries covered under the contracted clients' plans, follow PPO/EPO utilization review provisions and

quality assurance and peer-review decisions, maintain his license, remain on the active staff of the hospital, and pay dues promptly.

4. The physician promises to refer to other members or facilities under contract with the client and to use quality of care as the primary consideration for referral.

5. The member consents to participate in PPO/EPO utilization and quality assurance programs.

6. The member agrees to keep legible medical records and to allow timely inspection and audit of data without violating patient confidentiality.

7. The term of the agreement is fixed, usually for one year.

8. The member may cancel the contract on 90 days' notice. The PPO/EPO can terminate a member for loss of state medical license, dismissal from the medical staff, an act of fraud, a serious criminal offense, failure to comply within 15 days of notice with the PPO/EPO rules, bylaws, or the terms of any client contract.

9. If a member is terminated early or is not renewed at the end of a contract cycle, the member may pursue a formal appeal to the membership committee and the board of directors.

10. The PPO/EPO and the physician each remain independent.

11. The organization and each member carry their own liability insurance coverage at agreed upon minimum limits.

12. The member agrees to have his name and other information listed in clients' benefit plan documents.

13. Arbitration may be used to settle disputes between the member and PPO/EPO.

14. The member agrees to pay an annual fee for uses as described by the PPO/EPO.

15. The physician must purchase stock from and resell it to the PPO/EPO.

16. The PPO/EPO is permitted to verify medical staff membership information and obtain quality assurance and utilization data from health care organizations.

17. The agreement contains standard general terms related to assignment, binding effect, severability, counterparts, waiver, modification, notices, and governing law and venue.

The addition of an "attorney-in-fact" agreement to the membership agreement is a highly recommended option. Under current laws and practices, a PPO/EPO can only serve as "messenger boy" in contract negotiations. When a potential client offers a contract with a fee schedule to the group, the group's contracting committee must present that exact fee schedule without comment to each PPO/EPO member for individual signature. No negotiating with the client by the contracting committee on the fee schedule is permitted, although all other parts of the contract are subject to modification. As you can imagine, this slows the entire contracting process to a snail's pace.

The easy and effective solution to this tedious process is an attorney-in-fact contract (AIF) with each of the PPO/EPO provider members. Upon joining the PPO/EPO and at annual renewal, each member is offered an opportunity to give PPO/EPO officers permission to bind the members to any contract fee schedule at or above a threshold level selected by the member.

Here is a verbatim explanation from one AIF contract:

> The mechanism of this PPO contract may be different from others which you have signed in the past. With this contract you are asked to select the minimum conversion fee schedule ("threshold fee") you are willing to accept for your services. The PPO will then market the program. You are automatically included in any contract which meets or is above the "threshold fee" you have selected. This "attorney-in-fact contract" keeps you in control of your fees, while at the same time allows the PPO to know the size and composition of the panel available at any given fee schedule. These rates are determined by you and other panel members when the fee-selection portion of this contract is completed.

> With this arrangement, a client who wants to contract with our PPO can review the composition of the panel available at different fee levels. Obviously, the more a client is willing to offer, the larger the panel. All providers whose threshold fees were at or below

the offered schedule would be included on the client's panel. On the other hand, a client's medical panel would not include those providers whose threshold fees were at levels above that offered by the client. Those providers who are included in the panel will be notified that the PPO has exercised its power of attorney and has entered into the contract on their behalf.

Those physicians who are not included in the panel will be informed of the fee schedule being offered. Then, if any provider wishes to make an individual decision to participate at the offered fee schedule, he/she would contact the PPO office and indicate a willingness to accept the fee schedule being offered, even though it was below their threshold fee. If the notice is timely, and the panel not closed, they would be included on the panel.

The AIF contract is much easier to administer because the "messenger boy" process has been replaced with a "fax-system" and the contracting committee knows in advance what the panel makeup will be at the fee schedule offered by a client. With the panel members' threshold fees in a computer, the client, also, can be informed what panel size and consistency is available at any given offered fee schedule. Modifications in the fee schedule can be made if the client wishes another panel mix. Using an AIF contract saves considerable time. Most contracts can be signed within 24 hours, allowing a client to start printing directories and arranging employee sign-ups. The physician panel member who is not included on the AIF contract should always have another chance to participate at the offered fee schedule.

You must involve a knowledgeable attorney in the preparation and use of any type of contract. Federal antitrust penalties for errors are significant.

8. Hold a strategic planning session. Within the first six months after the PPO/EPO has been established, a strategic planning session should be held. When the board is ready for this important meeting, a formal mission statement should be prepared and distributed with the notice and other materials for the planning session. This session will develop a consensus among the membership about what the PPO/EPO is, its organizational strengths and weaknesses, where it wants to go during the next year, in three years, and in five years, and what it must do to get there. Strategic planning is an effort to direct or pull the membership into a common direction. It enhances membership education with the development of a common understanding of terminology, a realistic appraisal of past and present trends, and a rational projection of future goals and objectives.

The session may be planned and put on by the board itself without outside help. Unfortunately, unless a particular board member has the requisite skills, this is not advisable and may produce a meaningless meeting. If the PPO/EPO has a symbiotic relationship with the hospital, the administration may help underwrite the costs of a professional facilitator. Otherwise the PPO/EPO should raise the necessary funds from its membership for this service. There are numerous people in this business, and by asking around, good recommendations can be obtained to fit a modest budget. The PPO/EPO secretary can do the paperwork and mailings.

A facilitator requires 60 to 90 days to prepare for a meaningful strategic planning meeting with detailed interviews of the PPO/EPO leadership and a sample of its members. A study of the marketplace and competition is undertaken, and background materials are prepared. The membership should be given ample notice of the session, and materials should be mailed in sufficient time for study. Pull out all the stops to get a heavy turnout for this meeting.

9. Begin the contracting process. Most clauses in the PPO/EPO contract from an insurance company or other payer are negotiable at the time the client wants the services of the group. Here are some areas of special concern:

• "Hold harmless" clauses, which shield the client from damages if the physician errs. If, however, the care was compromised by utilization review decisions, it would seem to protect the client. If possible, eliminate this clause.

• The utilization review appeal process usually leaves the ultimate decision with the medical director of the review company.

Try to change this to your PPO/EPO or to a committee of your local medical society. The level of care rendered in one community may be significantly different from another. Local review standards are more appropriate.

• Most contracts will not allow a single group to have an exclusive contract within a community. If your group is of significant size and can adequately cover the needs of the client, an exclusive contract is worth seeking, even if the fee schedule is tightened a bit.

• Automatic contract renewal at the end of the initial contract period prevents the group from renegotiating the fee schedule in a timely manner. The termination date should be agreed upon and preceded by a 90-day period during which the terms can be reevaluated and rewritten if needed.

• Some clients may specify how much professional liability insurance members must carry. If your membership agreement specifies lower limits, you may be able to negotiate the contract limit downwards. If several contracts insist on a higher level of insurance than the PPO/EPO requires, the board of directors may want to review this amount and propose an increased standard to the membership.

• Many insurers delay payment to physicians as long as possible in order to capture the "float," which means they earn interest on that money as long as they hold it before paying the physician. The PPO/EPO contract will specify how soon after a completed claim is received by the payer that it is required to pay the fee. A 30-day limit is appropriate. Any longer is excessive and should be renegotiated. Ask if electronic billing would speed payment and, if it would, the group may want to develop this as a membership service.

Several other clauses should be viewed with caution, and the best advice on them is available from your attorney.

10. Establish public relations and marketing. The membership should receive communication from the PPO/EPO at least every two months, and monthly if possible. A newsletter permits the board and its committees to communicate significant information. Items for this newsletter would be the signing of new contracts, renewal or renegotiation of old contracts, changes in membership services, new members, meetings, and general announcements. It should be attractive, well-written, and informative. A graphic designer can prepare the logo and design at a nominal cost.

The marketing of PPO/EPO services is often coordinated with the marketing department of the hospital. The effort focuses on direct mail contact with new residents, placement of advertising, and marketing to potential client groups, such as self-insured companies and benefit consultants. Many hospitals mail material to new residents in the hospital catchment area, the region from which the hospital's clientele is drawn, and they usually are willing to add the PPO/EPO's material to the mailing. The hospital may underwrite the cost of a joint brochure. The wisdom of this will depend on how closely the group wants to be aligned and identified with the hospital. A brochure describing the group is a good marketing piece for members to place in their office lobbies and for distribution at meetings. It conveys to the public that the physician is involved in cost control and is a member of a larger group of physicians of many specialties that provides total, high-quality health care.

Direct advertising of the group through newspapers or in the Yellow Pages is a local issue. What works in one location may fail in another. A physician referral service has been successful in attracting new patients to the group. The committee should be given a budget to test some of these approaches before making any major commitments.

The local newspaper is a good place for a feature article on the development of the group. The spokesman quoted in the article perhaps should be the secretary or the hospital administrator to avoid the appearance that any single physician is being promoted.

The committee may want to develop a speakers panel and solicit opportunities to present informational programs to local business and service organizations. These groups are always seeking new subjects, and with the current concerns about spiraling health costs, a new medical entity is a worthwhile subject for a 30-minute talk. Speakers must be well prepared with slides and brochures or other materials, because a poor presentation is worse than none at all.

Direct marketing to local businesses for exclusive contracts is a joint effort for the public relations and contract review committees. Self-insured companies are the best initial targets. An introduction to the chief executive officer or the chief financial officer by a PPO/EPO member is the surest way to start discussions. Other targets are third-party administrators and benefit consultants who handle self-insured clients. Your membership should be an excellent source of referrals for direct marketing and contracting.

11. Create membership services. If the PPO/EPO is organized as a nonprofit entity, the rationale for attracting bids from vendors is the group's combined purchasing power. A group of even 20 physicians can command a discount on purchased services, such as paper goods, office supplies, health insurance, and telephone answering services. Some travel agents will give a special group rate if all travel purchases are funneled through their offices.

If the group is a for-profit corporation, the benefits of membership services take on new value because the group can realize a profit from the sale of these services. The committee is limited only by its imagination and enterprise in putting together packages of beneficial membership services. Centralized billing benefits all members almost immediately. With all billings made through a single office, the group has the added benefit of collecting valuable utilization data about its own members. Bills can be forwarded to payers electronically, thereby increasing accuracy and cash flow. Telephone answering services can be wholly purchased from or co-ventured with existing firms. The group may purchase its own nursing home or home health agency. An imaging center, mammography unit, recovery care facility, clinical laboratory, or other related medical facility can be partially or totally owned, with the profits underwriting operations of the group or plowed back into other investments.

A final word of caution: Physician-owned enterprises must set an example within the community for quality of care and efficiency of service. The public has little sympathy for the greedy physician who trades the public trust for mere economic gain.

But the physician has the right, and even the responsibility, to compete with hospitals and other entrepreneurs in the development and management of medical facilities. Against hospitals, our collective advantage is the ability to improve the efficiency of operations; against non-medical entrepreneurs, it is our dedication to the quality of patient care. Therefore, members of the PPO/EPO group should not back away from the investment opportunities they know best and are able to utilize in their patient care.

HARVEY E. KNOERNSCHILD, M.D., M.Med.Sci., was educated at the University of California, Berkeley (A.B.), and the University of California School of Medicine, San Francisco (M.D.). He completed his surgical residency at Ohio State University (M.Med.Sci.) under Dr. Robert Zollinger. He completed a tour of duty in the U.S. Public Health Service in colon cancer research for the National Cancer Institute. He has served on the founding board of directors of four PPO/EPO/IPA groups and is past president of South Bay Medical Group of San Jose, California. He holds an appointment as clinical associate professor of surgery, Stanford University School of Medicine. He is a Diplomate of the American Board of Surgery and a Fellow of the American College of Surgeons. Dr. Knoernschild has lectured widely on "Health Care Trends: The Second Industrial Revolution." He is the founder and editor of "CE/Q Medical Newsletter," a monthly publication dedicated to cost-efficiency and quality-enhancement. Dr. Knoernschild practices general surgery in San Jose, is active with the Rotary Club of San Jose, and serves on the board of directors of the San Jose Symphony. He is available to consult in the areas of preferred provider group development and contracting, and cost-efficiency in medicine.

14

Utilization Review
In Your Community

William Sueksdorf, M.D.

Professional Claims and Utilization Review of California (PRO-CURE) is a statewide managed health care service formed in 1986 when a group of Santa Clara County physicians created a limited partnership. PROCURE performs inpatient and outpatient utilization review, case management, claims audit, and a variety of tailored cost-management services for the insurance industry and self-insured clients.

The founders of PROCURE knew that health care costs were escalating beyond the rise in the consumer price index, and they identified a genuine market need. The physicians were willing to take a financial and emotional risk, because they knew that the success or failure of PROCURE would be impossible to disguise. It took courage for them to venture into the business side of medicine and create a different image for themselves within the local medical community. The risk has paid off. Now in its fourth year, PROCURE is generating significant revenue and has firmly established itself as a prototype for successful local review services nationwide.

Medicine has always been a science and an art. During the last two decades it has become something more—big business. I say this with a sense of regret because I entered practice at a time when physicians seemed secure in their expectation that they would earn a comfortable income providing quality care while devoting only modest attention to billing and collecting their fees. Unfortunately, this is no longer true.

I was first exposed to the forces changing the nature of health care as an inpatient psychiatric service administrator for a hospital in San Jose, California. As I participated in budget meetings in the late 1970s, it became increasingly clear that hospitals were in trouble. Throughout this century hospitals had been operating merely as workshops for physicians, with a simplistic formula of setting charges to assure only that revenues exceeded expenses. Hospitals had no particular interest in the relative merits of intensive care units or emergency room trauma capabilities other than to match community needs with hospital resources. A money-losing service that was needed and supported by the medical staff would be subsidized by fees from other billable services. If a hospital fell short of revenue projections, it merely restructured its daily charges. That quaint approach clearly was doomed.

Led by the entitlement programs of Medicare and Medicaid, third-party payers began changing the rules of the game. Hospitals were reimbursed according to their costs, with many non-patient care items excluded. In the short run, more of these costs were passed on to the privately insured. The difference between full fees and cost-based fees widened, and hospitals' daily rates skyrocketed. Public and private sector outlays were spiraling out of control, and the health care system confronted for the first time a barrage of efforts to fix the problem.

I was introduced to utilization review through my local medical society, which asked me to serve on a panel of psychiatrists helping a professional standards review organization create "peer review standards." These standards were written guidelines for individuals reviewing the necessity of hospitalization and continued inpatient care for all medical and surgical specialties. At our first meeting, we argued the merits of the concept ("It's not appropriate for anyone but the treating physician to answer the question of medical necessity.") and reflected upon the complexity of creating such standards given the reality that someone else would write them if we didn't ("If we don't do it, it will be done poorly by someone who doesn't understand the issues involved").

There was no prototype for our group. Santa Clara County physicians and hospitals had pioneered many innovations in medical practice, and this may have contributed to our group's perseverance. We emerged with standards, content that ultimately the "rightness" of medical decisions would be defended by competent clinicians and all would be well. We envisioned a clinically knowledgeable individual reviewing charts and determining whether criteria had been met for hospital admission or continued stay. When questions arose, the reviewer would discuss differences with the admitting physician. When complexities were involved, we envisioned appropriately trained clinicians discussing with peers the merits of treatment decisions.

Utilization review began affecting my inpatient practice in 1978. California officials had identified my hospital as having excessive admissions and patient days. I thought this was easily explained because a nearby state hospital had moved 3,000 adults suffering severe mental illness into licensed and unlicensed board and care homes within walking distance of our emergency room. We were confronted by a high daily volume of severe psychotic episodes, suicide attempts, and behavior that endangered others. Surely, we thought, this information would account for our "abnormal profile" and lead the reviewers at MediCal, California's Medicaid program, to make allowances for our special circumstance.

But MediCal was not interested in our problems. The state had set out to limit patient days, and utilization review was the tool to achieve that. A MediCal official came to our hospital and began making drastic decisions regarding medical necessity. "We're not telling you to discharge the patient," he said. "We're just telling you we won't pay beyond this date." I was appalled by such arbitrary, insensitive, and unqualified decisions. We were treating more severely ill county residents than any other private facility, and yet within three months our average length of stay had been reduced from the county norm of 12 days to 3.8 days. Our readmission rate was alarmingly high. Incredibly, the state's review system had no practicing psychiatrists involved in the review decisions or appeals.

This system ultimately led to a series of predictable and tragic outcomes. Doctors grew reluctant to attend to patients they couldn't adequately treat within four days. The hospital sustained greater bad debt losses as many patients entered the hospital without proof of eligibility and were released before such documentation could be obtained. The hospital's reputation suffered as we discharged disturbed patients in a marginally improved mental condition. By the end of 1980 it was clear that the unit could no longer operate, and it closed for financial reasons.

I took from this experience a keen awareness of the potential consequences of the misapplication of utilization review. It was not what our committee had feared, which was that one psychiatrist would tell another what's best for a patient he or she had never met. This was worse—a health care system using unqualified personnel applying unwritten guidelines for the sole purpose of reducing admissions and patient days. Still, I didn't see the bigger picture, and at the time I thought that this was just another indictment of MediCal ineptitude, not a reflection of practices one would encounter in the private sector.

Enter the private sector and its variation of utilization review. I can't say I remember my first telephone message to call Dr. so-and-so at an 800 number about one of my patients. In fact, it's likely that I wasn't calling a doctor at all, but a non-physician reviewing the medical necessity of an admission. By the early 1980s I was receiving such calls regularly. Someone in Ohio or Washington, D.C., or some other place far removed from my world would ask my estimate of the length of stay of an admitted patient and authorize a certain number of days for the diagnosis and condition I described. I found the calls to be an inconvenience, but I tolerated them as necessary. At the time, I still believed that, when all was said and done, reviewers would perceive the need for treatment if the physician communicated adequately.

As the months rolled by, more organizations began employing forms of review, and I remember thinking, "When is somebody going to do it right?" Here we were in the mid-1980s, a decade after my first involvement with the crafting of utilization standards, and the reviews remained a thorn in my side, distracting me from my patients and constantly reminding me that if I did not perform, the financial burden could be shifted from the payer to the patient.

I began seeking opportunities to move to the other end of the system. I became a psychiatric consultant for both Humana and Maxicare, working within their organizations to establish written guidelines and to insure that denials of coverage would be rendered concurrently with treatment and only by qualified psychiatrists. My involvement with these organizations helped me understand the managed care utilization review process, but I could see that my influence was extremely limited. I felt there wasn't much potential to make a difference.

This brought me to the verge of medical entrepreneurship. I could see that cost containment and cost management represented a new and permanent reality and that they would continue to grow as health care costs continued to spin out of control. Utilization review would play a major role in the foreseeable future, I believed, and because it was not being done well, there was the potential to create a new business: a professional review organization in which competently trained clinicians and allied health professionals set policies and applied standards appropriate to their geographic area. I just wasn't sure whether I had the courage to put time and financial resources into such a project.

What type of business was best suited for me? Was I really attracted to utilization review, or would I be more comfortable putting together a preferred provider organization? If I set up a psychiatric review service, how big would it need to be to conduct business? Would it be an advantage or disadvantage to operate as a stand-alone product? How long would it take? Would the time commitment force me to give up patient care? And if I did that, within a short time wouldn't I become unqualified to make review decisions by virtue of my increasing distance from the realities of everyday practice?

I didn't want to enter into a business whose decisions I could not influence, so I suspected I would need to be a sole owner, a partner, a board member, or a high-ranking administrator. I really wasn't sure which. I wanted to stay in the area of my expertise, mainly adult psychiatry, and I knew I was willing to invest significantly in myself if I could see the business was suitably structured. The notion of investing in my own business ideas was far more attractive than investing through an independent broker in a business involving people I had no knowledge of or control over.

The solution came unexpectedly from an organization called PROCURE. I had been contacted by a respected local surgeon who was looking for a psychiatrist to perform utilization review for a company he was forming. I expressed an interest in participating, and he asked me to submit a proposal. A variety of local physicians had pooled their talents to create a professional claims and utilization review organization with qualified professionals rendering decisions in their areas of expertise. They had anticipated the need to extend the concept to all health care services, including outpatient visits, dental care, pharmacy services, and home health care. I was very excited.

Foremost among my concerns about the structure of the business was the integrity and accountability of the decision-makers. As soon as I met the group that was being assembled into the board of directors, I knew this would not be an issue. These were all well-established, well-respected community clinicians, actively practicing their specialties. They all had experience with utilization review gone awry and were confident they could do it better. To my good fortune, they had not yet included mental health services, and I was a good fit for their group.

Had this opportunity not emerged, I doubt I would have independently pursued utilization review as a business chiefly because of my fear of committing the financial resources and personal time to an endeavor that could fail. I also knew that inadequate funding might lead to corner-cutting, a path taken by many existing utilization review companies. For example, some use poorly trained or unqualified staff members to make telephone decisions for geographic regions with which they have no familiarity. Despite having successfully operated a small business, my psychiatric practice, I felt my business background would be insufficient for me to take on such a project without significant help from business partners.

The PROCURE group had already identified its market: health care purchasers who wanted to control costs, such as self-insured employers or administrators of union trust funds. When we researched the available products and "ran some numbers" on business anticipated from these potential clients, an encouraging picture emerged. We figured it would be possible to create a substantial investment opportunity and capitalize the business through the formation of a limited partnership.

The major consideration at the start-up was predicting the costs of forming the partnership and operating the business until it could turn a profit. We believed that legal and accounting fees would be major expenses but that they were necessary to structure the partnership properly. We projected that a business could be conducted on a bare-bones budget until significant accounts were brought on board that required the hiring of more people. We also felt that if the concept proved successful in Santa Clara County, we could duplicate the program in adjacent counties through a franchise approach in which the general partners could pursue new groups of limited partners in noncompeting markets. Such a system eventually could cover the entire state. Clearly, it was crucial for us to obtain legal and tax advice so the entity could be organized to allow that growth.

The board decided to move ahead with the venture as a limited partnership. The general partner would become PROCURE, Incorporated, a California corporation with six practicing physicians and one insurance professional as owners and board members. The general partner would receive shares based on capital contributions. The organizers decided it was desirable to have each owner of the general partner begin with an equal interest in the corporation.

The limited partnership was seen as a vehicle to capitalize the business and strengthen its resources by inviting qualified health professionals to participate. While it was clear that not all our reviewers would invest, nor would all of our investors be reviewers, a significant number would do both. We felt this would give us a core of committed reviewers at a time when low case volume might make it difficult to retain those only interested in percase remuneration.

Our financial projections were very encouraging and we perceived that the major threat to success would be undercapitalization or overspending prior to the launch. We were confident that once we found customers, our profit margin would give us security. Our largest expense and the one that proved most difficult to control was legal fees. But I knew that the worst nightmare would be to establish a business and find out later that the corporate structure violated securities laws and the entire operation was in jeopardy. That not only could ruin a business, but it could tarnish the reputations of the people sponsoring it. It was clearly not a time for do-it-yourself or cut-rate legal aid. I believe that our lack of familiarity with the task before us led to mushrooming legal fees. There are many things to learn, and the meter runs at a steady rate. Great expense can be incurred whenever board members are confused about the directions given to the lawyers. All board members should understand the structure of the business and the legal implications of the offer of a limited partnership. Clarifications of the difference between the general partner, the limited partners, PROCURE, and PROCURE, Incorporated made it difficult to determine for which entity legal work was being performed and who was to be billed for it.

Limited partnerships can certainly be attractive investments, but they do not sell themselves. Determining that the investor is fully qualified and aware of the potential risks requires great effort. We had set a goal of capitalizing our business by selling $180,000 worth of limited partnership shares. These were to be achieved by selling 20 partnership interests at $9,000 each. Because we wanted to conclude our partnership offering within 120 days, we called a meeting at a local hotel and invited prospective investors to learn about the business concept. We distributed a prospectus and invited them to ask questions.

The meeting seemed successful. Our peers were quite positive, and many indicated they would be interested in participating either as investors or reviewers. Other potential investors said they would need to think about it. It appears in retrospect that we may have damaged our efforts by losing our focus.

Because we had allowed ourselves up to four months to close the sale of limited partnerships, I think the remote deadline lulled us into a lack of concern about sluggish sales. As the weeks wore on, we found that many people who said they would be willing investors had not submitted their paperwork or their money and that many of these follow-ups were handled in too casual a fashion. In the meantime, our business began to incur legitimate expenses, and we had to consider additional funding to tide us over until the limited partnership funds were collected and then became available.

The board of directors, having already capitalized a good deal of the start-up with their own money, decided that a line of credit would be the best source of additional funds. This was a tangible statement of the commitment and confidence that board members held regarding the viability of the business. Seeing the founding members demonstrate their willingness to back their venture with personal resources solidified our resolve to succeed.

Despite the discouraging initial collection of funds, prospective investors continued to give us positive feedback about the venture. As the deadline drew closer, we pursued the funds with new focus and energy and closed the limited partnership sales within the 120-day period, and eventually we raised $210,000. I see now that the same goal could have been reached with a more intensive sales effort initially. Were we to do this again, I would promote more uniform communication with potential limited partners.

We had emphasized our desire to maintain good relationships with our limited partners, but as is often the case, we had no plan to insure that this happened. The board soon recognized the need for regular communication with the limited partners, both in periodic meetings and in writing. At that point, the board decided to publish a newsletter to inform the investors about company activities. I was appointed editor.

The newsletter became an example of how a start-up company can at times take a concept and struggle with it for an extended period before settling on the exact nature of its final product. In my mind the newsletter was a vehicle to communicate with our limited partners about their investment. But it became clear that given the expense of producing and distributing a newsletter, it should serve as a marketing tool as well. The initial mailing was envisioned as a blanket approach aimed at potential customers as well as reviewers and our own investors. We called the publication "Review Matters" and assigned our internal staff to develop a format and graphics to save time and money. We wanted to publish as soon as possible. After completing our first publication and disseminating it to more than 500 individuals, we realized that we had not produced material that our investors needed to keep abreast of our progress.

We saw this lack of focus many times in our first two years. We would identify a project with a particular goal and find several other unmet needs along the way. The project would be changed mid-stream to meet what we felt was a greater and more urgent need and we ultimately would fail to achieve the initial goal. It is important for start-up companies to bear in mind the process of reviewing how a project started, what it ended up producing, and whether the original goal has been met. We ultimately solved our problem by decentralizing the process so that the full board was not needed for every decision. Committees proved helpful in solving this problem.

After PROCURE closed its limited partnership offering and hired a nucleus of employees and equipment, business began. The board met monthly to review company activities and attend to operational matters. We shared a temporary space of 1,600 square feet in an office building.

The first order of business was sales. In support of our marketing team, board members made themselves available to address groups and health care decision-makers for breakfasts, lunches, and any other meetings we could work into their schedules. We knew potential clients would be interested in our results and a list of current clients. Anxious to produce satisfied clients so we could give the right response to these questions, we tailored stand-alone products that we thought would attract individuals willing to try us on an introductory basis. We won some general review accounts, but our first big success came with a dental review contract. A company with a dental plan asked us to review bills submitted on covered members. The dentist making the review determinations was particularly familiar with codes and frequency of services, and he could identify when people were billing improperly and excessively.

We learned from our sales contacts that many companies wanted cost management but expected a slightly different product than what we were offering. At this point, about three months into our operation, we began a yearlong product development effort. It seemed as if every week or two our staff conceived a new product we could offer, and I can see now that this may well have been a problem to avoid. We wound up creating so many products (utilization review of inpatient and/or outpatient, with our without a gatekeeper, with or without a preferred provider organization, including or excluding chiropractic, podiatric, and mental health, etc.) that we could not describe any of our services in a simple fashion. Proposal writing became a headache because each one was a unique experience. A narrative text for one plan would not fit the next, and product pricing became a separate, cumbersome step in each proposal.

We developed a number of products, but after dropping some, we wound up with a menu of six identifiable services. It was demanding work, but our confidence was bolstered by the accounts we did sell. Utilization review, we found, could be performed effectively—we knew it all along! In our first few quarters we built our credibility with prospective clients by producing excellent results, defined by measurable savings to our customers. This gave the staff more ammunition for the sales attack, and after nine months we saw signs of moving into the black.

But then the marketplace gave us some new cues. Many of the businesses we had perceived as strictly local were actually operating with satellite groups across the state. They were only interested in buying our utilization review if we could handle all of their employees and dependents, a much more difficult task than working on smaller contracts. That service required either a long-distance review process—the very creature that had annoyed so many of us before—or the development of a statewide network.

PROCURE's founders knew from the beginning that the concept of local review was the most appropriate and that if the concept succeeded in Santa Clara County, it could be replicated in the form of local review services throughout the state. This was a rigorous test of our commitment to the original local review philosophy, and the board decided not to sacrifice it. The best review, we knew, would be peer-to-peer.

The marketplace had identified a need for a review group operating all over California, and while some organizations were providing that service, they invariably used out-of-state telephone review contacts or subcontracting with a wide variety of review entities—some well regarded and others quite inferior. This opportunity required a response that would maintain the integrity of our operation.

We worried that if we franchised our business by selling new limited partnerships in adjacent counties, we would be distracted by a series of fund-raising efforts throughout the state. In Santa Clara County alone it had taken us nearly six months to market the limited partnerships. An alternative that would not require major organizational efforts involved redefining the scope of our business and changing the name from "PROCURE of Santa Clara County" to "PROCURE of California." By redefining our business, we abandoned the original concept of separate limited partnerships in each county in California. Instead, we developed groups of reviewers in the major counties, with each group being linked to the company directly. In essence, we achieved the same end result: a network of local review panels responsible for doing the utilization review for our clients within their own medical communities.

The board decided to go ahead with the statewide plan, and we sent letters to the limited partners explaining why our expansion plan would be financially beneficial. Limited partners who wanted to avoid dilution of their accounts could purchase additional limited partnership shares up to the amount they currently held. The limited partners overwhelmingly endorsed the plan.

We identified the geographic areas that needed a full constellation of reviewers and began searching for key individuals to organize the local programs. It was our tenth month of operation, and we were pleased to see that our reputation was growing and plenty of contacts were "in the pipeline."

At that point, the press took an interest in PROCURE. The San Jose Business Journal featured a product called CDRx, for chemical dependency prescription, which we developed by networking our product with a local entrepreneur. The product combined our utilization review component with the existing employee assistance and intervention program and contracted facility/provider discounts. The Business Journal found CDRx newsworthy because of its cost-saving potential and because of the human interest in the subject of chemical dependency. We saw a spurt in activity in this product that assisted our sales people in landing several attractive contracts. This welcome media attention did not come accidentally. It was the result of working with a reporter contact who was seeking "newsworthy" items in health care for publication.

At the end of the first year of operations as a limited partnership, we had firm contracts and business on the horizon that would put PROCURE into the black. Sales still had been predominantly based in Santa Clara County, but we had decided to pursue the statewide market, and today we are extremely optimistic about the growth potential. The decision to expand increased our expenditures and delayed the start of profitability, but our investors continue to give us strong backing.

I believe this project could be duplicated outside of California. The concept of local review is more than just palatable to the clinicians—it offers the most rational approach to utilization review. Should such a concept indeed become a standard, demand will grow for local review groups to subcontract with larger groups, including national organizations. This may create additional opportunities for physicians who want to limit their business activities to their home regions. The key to success is the organization's commitment to use appropriately trained and qualified individuals to monitor decisions affecting health care cost management.

To those who question whether physicians should be involved in projects that are more business than medicine, I can only say that the two disciplines are not only compatible, they are synergistic. Those who go into PROCURE-style projects will gain a better appreciation of the new role of physicians in health care and see positive results in the care they render in their own practices.

WILLIAM SUEKSDORF, M.D., received his B.A. (chemistry, physics, and mathematics) from Whittier College, and his M.D. from the University of California School of Medicine, San Francisco (1973). He completed his internship and two years of psychiatric residency at the University of Oklahoma Hospital. His residency was completed at Stanford University, where he served as medical director of the psychiatric evaluation unit of the Palo Alto, California, Veterans Administration Hospital. Dr. Sueksdorf has been the medical director of the Hillview Methadone Clinic and of the Monte Villa Hospital of Morgan Hill, California. He is a faculty consultant for the family practice program at San Jose Medical Center and a lecturer for the Stanford University physician assistant program. He is active in the Santa Clara County Psychiatric Society and the Northern California Psychiatric Society. Dr. Sueksdorf practices in San Jose, California, and is consultant for Behavioral Health Associates on the Conditional Release Program. He is available as a consultant in the area of psychiatric and chemical dependency utilization review.

15

The Planning and Design
Of a Health Facility

Paul Schrupp, B.A.

A giant relief map is mounted on the wall at the Sacramento headquarters of the California Association of Hospitals and Health Systems. On it, each of California's 550-plus hospitals is represented by a pushpin. The hospital association staff has taken great care to color code the pushpins on the map. One color is for privately-owned hospitals, another for the non-profits, and the remaining colors stand for various governmental entities, such as district, Veterans Administration, county, and university hospitals.

This color-coded scheme of health delivery is most striking in two-hospital towns. There are a surprising number of them in California. They are typically small farming communities in the Central Valley that have been insulated from the state's growing urbanization. On the map, these towns are small enough for one pushpin to overshadow the entire city limits, leaving the second to stake out some nearby cotton field or walnut orchard. Invariably the pins that nudge each other for the same piece of rural topography are never the same color. One of the pins must always represent the non-profit hospital that was established by the city's forefathers back in Clara Barton's day, while the competitor is linked to a large hospital chain.

Over the years, the two facilities almost certainly have bickered about various projects and community issues. Their quarreling has always revolved around the one anxiety both facilities share: that the medical staff is abandoning them to participate in the competitor's latest venture. With this phobia hanging on the wall of their board rooms, which of these hospitals would ever fail to hire an administrator who couldn't roll up the shirtsleeves, put on an "all ears" look, and manage the concerns and complaints of the medical staff with a smile bright enough to win a congressional seat?

Having grown used to the verbal massage, the physicians had become indifferent to administrators or the battles they have to wage. A decade ago, the certificate of need program allowed for remote skirmishes that only seemed to involve the two hospitals. Each would take turns flying expensive lawyers up from the "Big City" to stand in a high school cafeteria and argue that the approval of some lengthy document would yield a great benefit to the local citizenry. The physicians could never understand the hospital's inability to get anywhere in the game, they did not particularly care for the use of lawyers, and for the most part, the process was too confusing to encourage their participation in hospital planning and marketing.

The advent of contract medicine thrust hospitals onto a new battleground. Certificate of need programs fell by the wayside, and among the first casualties were health planners and the "all ears and little action" school of hospital administration. Physicians generally got their first exposure to this game when the administrator of one of the local hospitals offered shares of stock in the facility's parent company. In return, the physicians were expected to give a 40-percent discount to a health maintenance organization that had contracted with the hospital. Physicians were not interested in participating, but they could see the day when their hospital patients would be regarded as second-class citizens due to the politics of nonalignment.

Imagine their surprise when the administrator of the community hospital approached them recently to explain that the hospital was purchasing a local medical practice to develop a "full-scale" primary medicine clinic, and he wanted them to invest in it. Not only were they turned off by the investment, but they were hardly excited about having to compete with the hospital's marketing department for their patients.

Yet rarely does the disaffection with local hospital politics spur physicians to develop their own enterprises. Strained relations are more often the backdrop. The initiative to develop a competing facility usually begins when the hospital administration's commitment to other non-patient programs stands ahead of physician requests to improve a patient-sensitive service. A critical mass is finally reached, and the practitioners stop grumbling about how things should be done and decide to do it themselves. In this sense, most physician enterprises are remarkably egotistic. The founding partners are not especially concerned about the financial aspects of a project, but rather they are seeking superior service for their patients. And they are confident they can provide it more effectively away from the hospital.

With a little organization, professional help, and a considerable supply of patience, most physicians have the skills to put together their own projects. The do-it-yourselfer should begin with the simple theorem that the success of every project is tied to utilization. This equates to the individual caseloads of the participating physicians. It is a mistake to begin a project with a battery of consultants preparing a business plan and multi-colored demographic charts. The first step is to find out how much interest local physicians have in seeing the new service available in the community.

This is best accomplished by face-to-face meetings with other physicians. Mailings and questionnaires are an inadequate means of gauging the medical community's sentiments. The organizers should be equipped with accurate financial projections, which demonstrate the profitability of the project at varying activity levels or caseloads. Those physicians who are most inclined to support the project should be approached first. If the project has strong support from the outset, it has a much greater chance of securing additional support down the road.

Although an option on a piece of land is not necessary, it's best to have a specific location in mind for the project. The importance of the site cannot be overstated, because a suitable location means convenience for the physician and the patient. It is a mistake to think that a physician will endure inconvenience merely because of an ownership interest in a project. Most people prefer not to climb into a car and drive extra blocks to hunt for parking places, and physicians are no exception. The assurance of universal convenience will greatly enhance the success of any medical facility.

The financial projections prepared for potential investors should not include extreme inflation assumptions. If the project is going to be successful, it should be successful in today's dollars and not rely on an inflationary trend to show profits. There are many non-economic factors that go into national health care charges and expenditures. Even if charges continue their upward spiral, there is no political assurance that Medicare and Medicaid programs will maintain funding consistent with those inflation levels. The incorporation of large across-the-board revenue inflators in financial projections can badly skew otherwise accurate figures.

Good financial projections are best obtained from someone who has experience in developing a similar project. Some accounting firms and financial analysts develop health facility financial projections with cost estimates based on commercial building cost indices. This is a serious mistake as the cost of developing a health facility is considerably higher than a commercial medical office building. Zoning often requires a conditional use permit, and municipal deliberations can drag on for months while issues like infectious waste and ambulance access are debated. Architectural fees for health care projects are higher because the specialized service requires more detail in working drawings. Structural safety requirements imposed on health facilities demand considerably higher engineering fees. The plan check review is usually longer and often involves more than four different governmental agencies.

When construction gets under way, initial site work is going to be more expensive because a health facility's structural standards compel a larger and more elaborate foundation. The shell costs are higher because of more stringent seismic, occupancy, and fire standards, not to mention the provision of additional services such as emergency power and piped medical gas. Interior tenant improvement costs are higher than in comparable commercial buildings because most health facilities require specialized equipment wiring and increased plumbing.

An exacting outline of the project's costs must be completed early in the development stage, so it might as well be the first item on the planning agenda. Projections of expenses and revenues should be consistent with similar facilities that provide the same service and should reflect the revenue base already existing in the community. When meeting with individual physicians to present the financial feasibility and secure their support, it is not necessary to have an offering circular or a formal organization. The project will come together on its own if there is sufficient community interest. If there isn't, there is little sense in proceeding any further.

The decision on how a project should be organized will frequently be a political, not an economic, decision. Each local situation is different, so there is no preferred format for organizing a physician enterprise. Many are successful as partnerships, and many are successful as corporations. Different people will look at the project with different interests. Some will want a strong say in the management, while others may wish to make a one-time investment and enjoy a quality service.

Usually, the interests of the participants, their personal financial resources and the type of project being developed determine the appropriate organizational structure of the business. Whichever legal structure is chosen, when investors are to be solicited to capitalize the project, the projected return should be conservative and the investment reasonable. Although it may be common for real estate syndications to give organizers high promotional fees, special purchase options, management agreements, and exceptional priority on returns, the syndication of a medical enterprise should be regarded as a long-term investment. If the enterprise relies on the operating expertise of the organizers, they should be adequately compensated for the extra risks and liabilities they incur above other partners or shareholders. And just as the project should reward them for performance, it should also penalize them for failure.

Once the organization is formalized, a financing strategy should be put together. One element to consider in this strategy is the separation of real estate and equipment ownership from health care operations. The separation of these entities may afford greater long-term flexibility as interests in the different entities can be financed or sold independently. As local real estate markets cycle independently of health care markets, there may be a future benefit in refinancing the building or even moving the project to a different site.

Whatever legal format is selected by the organization, initial capitalization is extremely important. The project should not only be able to open its doors with a small contingency margin, but it should be able to remain in business for several months after the opening with little or no income. A new facility's accounts receivable always seem larger than anticipated. It takes time for insurance carriers to plug a new provider into their reimbursement network, and it takes time for the facility's billing staff to orient themselves to the billing procedures of a new set of payers.

The financing should be evaluated objectively. Despite the fact that everyone knows a great banker who promises to eliminate red tape, lenders are selling a product. As such, they should meet the same objective criteria imposed on an equipment vendor. In addition to commercial banks, credit lenders such as large corporations and life insurance companies should be explored as potential financing resources. In areas where the bulk of a project's labor will be performed by union tradesmen, union pension trusts should be evaluated as a source of financing.

Each prospective lender should be asked to submit a proposal prior to the submission of a loan application. The proposal should detail (1) the lender's experience with that type of project, (2) who will handle the loan, (3) the precise documents required, and (4) the conditions under which the loan will be approved. The proposal should include the loan rate and a complete schedule of loan costs, including title and legal fees. If legal fees are unknown because arrangements with the construction lender have yet to be established, a cap on legal fees should be considered. The schedule should indicate which of the costs can be financed with proceeds from the loan. Each lender should also be asked to indicate the number of days it will take to issue a committment letter once the application is approved, and the number of days it will take to close the loan once the commitment letter is given.

Unless one lender will be providing both permanent and construction financing, the permanent, or "take-out," loan should be established first. This reduces the construction lender's risk, and consequently the rate. The timing of the take-out is important. Permanent financing that activates upon issuance of the occupancy permit is the most desirable, whereas a "takeout" after two years or upon the attainment of a particular level of occupancy is less desirable. The lender that submits the second best proposal should always be advised of its standing, and copies of all application documents should be prepared in the event the first lender falls through. Even in the best of circumstances, this is a remarkably common occurrence.

A floor plan should be developed that minimizes non-revenue producing space and still balances aesthetic and operational needs. Because of the high cost of constructing a health facility, unused floor space such as corridors and storage spaces are kept to a minimum. The space plan is developed from four axes: patient flow, staff flow, materials flow and equipment siting.

Patient flow is a natural progression that keeps incoming patients from encountering exiting patients. Patient privacy is always an important consideration. If patients are expected to converse at the check-in area or during a consent explanation or examination, their conversations must not be easily overheard by others. Rest rooms are conveniently located near changing areas, lab areas, or wherever patients or family members may be subjected to long waits. If patients are to be discharged in wheelchairs to waiting automobiles, the roof of the discharge area protects them from the weather.

The staff should be able to enter and exit the facility without crossing through patient areas. Staff lounges and offices are out of earshot from patient areas. Sterile areas do not impede access to remote areas by the office staff and others who are not gowned. Wherever practical, the staff should not be split up. It is often convenient for one person to float between patient care areas following peak demands; this arrangement is most practical when nursing and supervisor stations are able to service separate patient areas.

The design of the materials flow starts at their point of entry into the facility. Outside access to the materials entrance is ample for large trucks, and, if necessary, curbs are ramped for hand trucks. The entrance way is restricted or monitored so that truck drivers do not wander into sterile areas looking for a signature to a delivery receipt. If possible, bulk storage areas are located at the materials entry to minimize handling, and to allow for immediate storage before unpacking and distribution. Without a convenient storage area, bulk supplies tend to be parked in corridors until they can be shelved.

The facility's supplies and materials are distributed internally to locations where they are most convenient for use. After supplies have been soiled, their progression to disposal or reprocessing follows a route that does not cross the flow of clean materials. Most health care facilities generate a considerable amount of trash, and for this reason, trash storage is convenient to any clean-up room. If a portion of the waste is potentially infectious, trash storage and handling areas must accommodate duplicate containers to permit the segregation of contaminated refuse. Trash storage areas must also be easy to wash down. Indoors, this generally requires a floor drain and a wall surface that is resistant to moisture. If the trash area is outdoors, and a drain is installed for washdown, most cities will require a roof to keep rainwater out of the municipal sewage.

Equipment siting is especially important. Electrical sub-paneling is conveniently placed so that the tripping of a breaker does not require a dark sojourn to the basement. Likewise, medical gas storage should allow quick access to a tank room without having to negotiate an undue number of locked doors. Compressors and other heavy equipment are located away from treatment areas. Their noise is bothersome, and even minor floor vibration can sharply restrict delicate tasks. Ventilation fans are located as close as possible to the air discharge registers. Health facilities maintain asepsis by using high air exchange ratios and heavy filtering. This requires large fans to move a high volume of air. The cost of the energy needed to move a large amount of air can be astronomical if the distance is not minimized.

It is best to bring the architect into the project early to assist in the development of the space plan. There are numerous basic guidelines for space design, particularly with corridors and exits. For the most part, architects are experienced with this task and can offer good insight. Before doing any work, the architect should bid the entire project against other qualified architects. The contract should include schematic drawings necessary for all municipal permits and approvals, complete construction drawings, submission of the drawings to building officials, supervision of the contractor's bidding, review of shop drawings submitted by outside vendors, certification of the contractor's applications for payment, and sufficient site visits to properly monitor the construction.

In many design-build situations, it will not be possible to bid the architect. Moreover, a developer-contractor will resist the notion of an architect administering the construction. These objections are usually prefaced with, "We don't need somebody to tell us how to build a building, now do we?" The architect is, however, your advocate and should be used to assure that you get what you paid for. Few lay people are competent to check the adequacy of caulking in a smoke partition or read an air balance report.

Experience is important when selecting an architect. In terms of costs, an architect who has designed several similar facilities will probably charge less than a large hospital-oriented architectural firm and will provide an equivalent, if not greater, amount of talent. The architect should break down his fees for the entire project and provide a schedule for outside consultants such as mechanical, structural, electrical, civil, kitchen, or landscape professionals.

If the architect is a temperamental artist with a priceless creative genius, this format will at least establish a value for the art work. Local architects tend to stress the importance of having someone who has worked with the local planning department. Their pitch may portray a city zoning code as so restrictive that special approval is needed just to put a handle on a mail box. Municipal planners, however, are accustomed to working with out-of-towners and are quick to point up the key elements of consideration.

If it is determined that only a local architect will understand the city's complicated solar power ordinance, a local architect could be used for the site and elevation drawings, and an experienced health facility architect employed to handle the overall project development. Architects are accustomed to working with each other in this capacity, and it does not cause confusion or unnecessary expense. Experience is more important than influence and should not be traded away for local political conditions. If influence is needed to present issues at the local level, a professional with the proper influence should be retained. Every city has an attorney who sat on the city council for six years and still plays tennis with the mayor.

The interior designer should be brought into the project soon after the architect. There are many decisions to be made in the course of construction that require the designer's input. It will not cost any more to bring the designer in early, and the results are better if the architecture and construction are coordinated with the interior motif. Both the architect and designer should be given a budget before they commence.

During the design phase of the project, it's important to remember that many costly features will seem worth the additional expense. It is best to list these extras as "adduct-alternatives." When the construction job is bid, the various contractors will price each of the alternatives, thus allowing an evaluation of the actual base cost as well as other extraordinary features that may be omitted from the final design for budgetary reasons.

Although many lease agreements will not permit a bidding process, it is preferable to have the general contractor bid the project. Those permitted to bid should have experience with health facilities, not just commercial medical office buildings. The bids should provide a list of subcontractors and their respective bids. The contractor should include a schedule for the completion of the project and the cost of a performance bond. The performance bond is insurance that the contractor will be in business at the completion of the project, and many construction lenders will require it as a loan condition. The imposition of liquid damages and the posting of a performance bond are a matter of preference and often depend on other circumstances. The bond has a cost associated with it, and the contractor can usually quote its dollar value.

If it is critical that the project be completed by a certain date, it may be prudent to impose a penalty for delays. The penalty, or liquid damages, is the contractor's liability if the project is not finished by the contracted completion date. A contractor will consider liquid damages at the time of the bid and thus bid higher if the penalty poses a significant risk. Liquid damages are usually minimal. The idea is not to impose harsh sanctions for unforeseen delays but to give the contractor a small incentive to stay on top of the subcontractors.

Before the architectural drawings can be completed, the project's fixed equipment plan must be developed. This is prepared as an itemized list that includes the data and specifications for all equipment required for the project's engineering, construction and operation. There are numerous equipment vendors that will organize the equipment plan if the client agrees to purchase the facility's equipment from them. No one in the health care business pays list price for equipment, especially if a large amount is being purchased at one time. For this reason, every vendor promises terrific discounts that are only possible because of "national purchasing agreements" or their "interest in a long-term relationship." If an independent consultant assists in equipment planning, it's preferable that he or she receive a set fee and allow commissions and savings to be passed directly through to the client. Equipment selection should be competitive.

The equipment plan must be thorough. It is not sufficient merely to provide specifications for all equipment. These specifications are summarized and made as easy as possible for subcontractors to read at the site.

Any piece of large equipment will require an orchestration of many events to assure that it is properly installed. An autoclave, for example, is little more than an oven required by most facilities to clean and sterilize equipment. To site a large unit in a specific room requires a considerable amount of detail. If it runs on 220 volts of electricity and the building has a 208-volt electrical service, a booster transformer will be required. If the autoclave is used to support an emergency service, it must be linked on a special circuit to the emergency generator. If it relies on a continuous supply of steam, a steam generator is needed. This in turn requires a steam filter, a pre-heater, and possibly a water softener. The autoclave, steam generator, and heaters require drain lines and condensate overflow lines. The power panels of all these items may require as much as three feet of clearance from walls and other equipment. Each of these units must be independently vented, and there may be a specific air exchange ratio for the rooms in which they are located.

Because equipment installation requires cooperation from numerous sub contractors, a good summary allows a quick look at the important details:

Item: X-ray illuminator

Manufacturer: General Electric

Model: E50887 AB

Vendor: General Electric Medical Systems
P.O. Box 414
Milwaukee, WI 53201

Description: Film illuminator. Dual (side by side). Surface mounted.

Size: 20 inches high, 30 inches long.

Finish: To be specified by designer.

Electrical: Provide 118 volt, 60 Hz, single phase 0.75 amps. Connect to emergency generator via critical care circuit.

Remarks: California seismic codes require a 1.5 importance factor. Contractor to ensure anchorage to code. Centerline of viewer to be 64 inches above floor; contractor to receive, unload, store, and set in place.

The equipment plan should provide for a delivery time, a delivery place, and a delivery procedure. Most vendors require 90 to 120 days to process orders for large specialty equipment. This must be coordinated with the construction schedule, and arrangements must be made to deliver and install. This is especially important if the equipment is very large or heavy. It is not uncommon to have delivery problems because a piece of equipment is too heavy for an elevator or is too large to be delivered through 42-inch doors. The equipment plan should have a receiving procedure to monitor delivery, and to make claims for equipment that may have been damaged during shipping.

Used or refurbished equipment can provide a significant savings if the purchaser is sufficiently familiar with the item to determine its value. If the large piece of used equipment will serve an important role in the facility's operations, a visit to the refurbisher's shop is highly recommended to see how their stock is overhauled. All bearings and plumbing lines are replaced. Movable parts such as hinges or gears are completely disassembled, inspected, and cleaned. Pneumatic cylinder assemblies are rebuilt, and electric motors rewound. Refurbished equipment must be purchased well in advance of the installation date to allow adequate time to order new equipment should refurbished items be unavailable. In this instance, arrangements must be made for storage until installation. Such storage should be in a location that is insured for loss or damage.

The movable equipment and instruments will be delivered shortly before the facility opens. Because the contractor does not install this equipment, the task of receiving it will be the responsibility of the facility's staff during their first days of service. Because this is always a hectic time, a receiving procedure is established to assure that relatively untrained personnel can assemble the equipment so it will be ready for immediate use. The contents of incoming parcels must be consistent with their packing slips, which in turn must be compared with invoices to verify the receipt of the items that were ordered.

The facility's staff should establish an inventory system that allows orderly stocking and monitoring of the disposable inventory. Because a new facility is purchasing its medical supplies with borrowed funds, it is especially important to keep the supply stocks to a bare minimum. The materials management system must work toward a "just-in-time" delivery of needed supplies.

Every facility should start with a skeleton staff and careful scheduling. It is not uncommon to begin with a caseload that is lower than anticipated. An idle staff can be very poor for employee morale, and extremely expensive to carry on a working capital loan. It is far better to open a facility that is understaffed rather than overstaffed. A layoff in the opening months can jeopardize staff loyalty for years to come.

The facility's opening date is coordinated with the various regulatory agencies and any final inspections that are required before patients can be received. To staff the facility and then delay the opening for two weeks to allow for corrections and reinspections can be very expensive. The agencies should be kept abreast of the project, and all paperwork in terms of policies and procedures is discussed with the regulators in advance. Procedure manuals are not necessarily acceptable for use in the new project just because they were acceptable elsewhere. Surveyors determine quality by the recording of a facility's events. They expect procedure manuals to be specific to the facility at hand and to be a cookbook for every activity. The facility with a system of procedures linked to logs and record-keeping will always appear to a surveyor to be superior to one that provides good medical care merely by policing its practitioners.

Several states require physicians to advise patients of their economic interest in an enterprise before a referral is made. This should be done irrespective of the legal requirement and presented in the positive light under which most physician investments are intended. If physicians commit personal resources to a project that delivers superior care and lower charges to their patients, they should be proud of it, and their patients should know how an important service came about.

One last important consideration before the ribbon-cutting is a full understanding of the price schedule. A common myth in medical enterprises is that physicians never know or care about a facility's charge schedule (this is only true if the price is lower than the competition's). Because physicians commonly handle price-related inquiries from either moderate-income patients who are uninsured or those who have 80-percent coverage, they should be aware of the financial impact on the patient. The facility's charges should cover the overhead, be fair to patients, and remain low enough to encourage physician referrals.

Low prices should never be advertised. A new facility must not try to compete on the basis of patient charges. In all likelihood, the local hospitals have the resources to withstand a price war. While keeping prices low, a new facility can best promote the issues that are important to physicians. Superior patient care and physician convenience will be used to market the facility. Lower prices will be a matter of private negotiation between the facility and organizations that refer patients solely on the basis of price, such as prepaid plans, clinics with capitated patients, and self-insured employer groups.

When the facility opens, a new community resource is born. For the two-hospital town, a third dimension is added to the scheme of health care delivery. The new enterprise always will have the option of linking services to the hospital of its choice. It also will be able to bargain with preferred provider organizations, HMOs, insurance carriers, and self-insured employee groups directly. Its ability to contain the cost of care will make it a stronger competitor when health care dollars become more scarce. As physicians opt to establish health care enterprises to protect the quality and independence of their practices, these free-standing flagships of low-cost, quality care may actually pin a few hospitals to the wall.

From the short-term perspective, this evolution cannot be regarded as a positive trend by the hospital industry. Physician enterprises have already been denounced as manifestations of physician greed, and competing hospitals are apt to increase this rancor as the struggle for shrinking health care resources continues. Proponents of institutional care are especially shrill with their allegations of "skimming," the so-called practice of accommodating the private paying patients while saddling hospitals with less profitable public patients.

After several decades of silence, however, physicians are once again taking an active role in shaping the health care system that revolves around their art. The growth of enterprises that provide cost-effective care and are well coordinated with physician practices cannot be regarded as a disaster to health care economies. Limited health care resources make it increasingly difficult to subsidize institutions that warehouse patients who could be cared for elsewhere. The physical plant and support services of a large hospital are inordinately expensive. As technical medical disciplines continue to advance with new equipment and procedures, it is not likely that these costs will decrease in the near future. Public and private payers must instead be encouraged to look to alternative resources that accommodate patients less expensively. Hospitals that survive this pressure will rely on the concentration of truly acute patients in acute settings, and employ appropriate linkages with alternative entities when superior care can be provided in a more cost-effective environment.

———————————

PAUL SCHRUPP is a graduate of the University of California at Davis (B.A.). He has been an associate with the independent consulting firm of Randlett Associates in Sacramento, California, for 12 years. Since joining the firm as a specialist in legislative and regulatory issues in the health care field, he has assisted the development of more than 20 health care facilities ranging from surgery centers to small hospitals. He is also the executive director of the Association of California Surgery Centers. He has served as an expert witness on surgery center issues and is a frequent speaker on surgery center development. Representing Fresno Recovery Care, he coordinated the passage of legislation permitting the development of 13 post-surgical recovery care facilities in California. This pilot project is the first of its kind in the nation, as it permits the overnight accommodation of post-surgical patients recuperating from major surgery in alternative hospital settings. Mr. Schrupp is available for consulting services.

Bibliography

Chapter 1

American Hospital Association Guide to the Health Care Field. Am Hospital, 1987.

Amodeo, Adele, et al. *Health Plan Design for California Non-Profit Organizations.* SF Study Ctr., 1985.

Callahan, James J., Jr., and Wallack, Stanley S., eds. *Reforming the Long-Term-Care System: Financial & Organizational Options.* Lexington Bks., 1981.

Culyer, A.J., and Horisberger, B., eds. *Economic and Medical Evaluation of Health Care Technologies* (Illus.). Springer Verlag, 1983.

Keets, Robert B., and Nelson, Mary. *The Medical Marketplace* (Illus.). Network Pubns., 1985.

Kett, Joseph F. *The Formation of the American Medical Profession: The Role of Institutions, 1780-1860.* Greenwood, 1980.

National Research Council and National Research Council Staff, *Profit Enterrise in Health Care.* Natl Acad Pr., 1986.

Schramm, Carl J., ed. *Health Care and Its Costs* (An American Assembly Book) (Illus.). Norton, 1987.

Snoke, Albert W. *Hospitals, Health and People.* Yale U Pr., 1987.

Chapter 2

American Medical Cost Effectiveness Plan: 1985 and Beyond. AMA, 1985.

Bloom, Harold. *The Hospital-Physician Relationship.* AHPI, 1986.

Brandt, Steven G. *Entrepreneuring.* Addison-Wesley Publishing Company, 1982.

Burns, Linda A., and Manacino, Douglas M. *Joint Ventures Between Hospitals and Physicians: A Competitive Strategy for the Healthcare Marketplace.* Dow Jones-Irwin, 1986.

Conway, Jennifer, ed. *Hospital Marketing,* rev. ed. L Davis Inst., 1986.

Drucker, Peter F. *Innovation and Entrepreneurship.* Harper & Row, 1986.

198

Eisenberg, John M. *Doctors' Decisions and the Cost of Medical Care: The Reasons for Doctor's Practice Patterns and Ways to Change Them*. Health Admin Pr., 1986.

Eller, Jack, ed. *Health Care Joint Ventures*. Rynd Comm., 1987.

Gladstone, David J. *Venture Capital Handbook*. Reston Publishing Company, Inc., 1983.

Hall, Craig. *Craig Hall's Book of Real Estate Investing*. Holt, Rinehart and Winston, 1982.

Jones, Deborah, et al. *A Guide to Assessing Ambulatory Health Care Needs in Your Community*. Abt Bks., 1974.

The New Health Care for Profit: Doctors and Hospitals in a Competitive Environment. Natl Acad Pr., 1983.

Peters, Tom. *Thriving on Chaos*. Alfred A. Knopf, 1987.

Peters, Tom, and Austin, Nancy. *A Passion for Excellence*. Random House, 1985.

Peters, Tom, and Waterman, Robert H., Jr. *In Search of Excellence*. Harper & Row, 1982.

Prack, Valencia N., et al., eds. *Health Care Ethics—Dilemmas, Issues and Conflicts*. Midwest Alliance Nursing, 1986.

Siafaca, Katie. *Investor Owned Hospitals and Their Role in the Changing U.S. Health Care System*. Ballinger Pub., 1981.

State Efforts at Health Care Cost Containment. Natl Conf State Legis., 1984.

Von Oech, Roger. *A Kick in the Seat of the Pants*. Harper & Row, 1986.

Von Oech, Roger. *A Whack on the Side of the Head*. Creative Think, 1984.

White, Richard M., Jr. *The Entrepreneur's Manual*. Chilton Book Company, 1977.

Chapter 3

Agich, George J., and Begley, Charles E., eds. *The Price of Health*. Kluwer Academic, 1987.

Ambulatory Medical Care Records: Uniform Basic Data Set Final Report. National Center for Health Statistics, 1974.

Anbar, Michael. *Computers in Medicine*. Computer Sci., 1987.

Avery, Maurine, and Imdieke, Bonnie. *Medical Records in Ambulatory Care*. Aspen Pub., 1983.

The Business Side of Medical Practice. AMA, 1986.

Cooper, Philip D., ed. *Responding to the Challenge: Health Care Marketing Comes of Age*. Am Mktg., 1986.

Cooper, Robert D. *Health Care Cost Management: Issues, Strategies and Current Practices; Final Report and Fact Book,* Brennan, Mary E., ed. Intl. Found. Employ., 1984.

Fein, Rashi. *Medical Care, Medical Costs.* Harvard U Pr., 1986.

Fox, Peter D., et al. *Health Care Cost Management: Private Sector Initiatives.* Health Admin Pr., 1984.

Goldfield, Norbert, and Goldsmith, Seth B. *Financial Management of Ambulatory Care.* Aspen Pub., 1984.

Goldsmith, Seth B. *Ambulatory Care: Theory and Practice.* Aspen Pub., 1978.

Laaser, U., et al., eds. *Primary Health Care in the Making* (Illus.). Springer-Verlag, 1985.

Moore, Anthony R. *The Missing Medical Test: Humane Patient Care.* Melbourne U Pr., 1978.

Sullivan, Sean, and Ehrenhaft, Polly. *Managing Health Care Costs: Private Sector Innovations.* Am Enterprise, 1984.

Chapter 4

Asfahl, Ray. *Industrial Safety and Health Management,* rev. ed. (Illus.). Prentice Hall, 1984.

Boley, Jack. *A Guide to Effective Industrial Safety.* Gulf Pub., 1977.

Brown, Marianne P. *A Worker's Guide to the Right to Know About Hazards in the Workplace.* U Cal LA Indus Rel., 1987.

Buchele, Maxine, and Wynn-Williams, Susan. *Successful Private Practice: A Guide to Effective Medical Practice Management.* Churchill, 1987.

Center for Occupational Research and Development Staff. *Agribusiness Safety.* Ctr Res and Dev., 1981.

Chadd, Charles M. *Practice Under the Occupational Safety and Health Act.* BNA, 1982.

Confidentiality of Patient Health Information. Am Med Record Assn., 1985.

Corbett, William A., ed. *Medical Applications of Microcomputers.* Wiley, 1987.

Creighton, Breen, and Gunningham, Neil, eds. *The Industrial Relations of Occupational Health and Safety.* Methuen Inc., 1985.

Encyclopedia of Occupational Health and Safety. Intl Pubns Serv., 1983.

Giordano, Daniel A. *Occupational Health Promotion: A Practical Guide to Program Development.* Macmillan, 1986.

Goldsmith, Frank, and Kerr, Lorin E. *Occupational Safety and Health: The Prevention and Control of Work-Related Hazards.* Human Sci Pr., 1982.

Joe, Barbara E., and Ostrow, Patricia C. *Quality Assurance Monitoring in Occupational Therapy.* Am Occup Therapy, 1987.

Labor and Employment Law ABA Section Staff, et al., eds. *Occupational Safety and Health Law.* BNA, 1987.

Maggart, Thomas A. *Cost Accounting: A Healthcare Management Tool.* Healthcare Fin Mgmt Assn., 1985.

Oberst, B.B., and Long, J.L. *Computers in Private Practice Management* (Illus.). Springer-Verlag, 1987.

Wallace, Stephen R., et al. *A Guide for Clinical Social Work in Health Care: New Biopsychosocial Approaches.* Praeger, 1984.

Yanda, Roman L. *Doctors as Managers of Health Teams: A Career Guide for Hospital-Based Physicians.* Bks Demand UMI.

Chapter 5

Ambulatory Health Care Standards Manual. Joint Comm. Hosp., 1986.

AORN, *Operating Room Staffing Study and Operating Room Cost Survey Report.* Assn. Oper. Rm. Nurses, 1984.

Center for Research in Ambulatory Health Care Administration Staff, and Lawson, James G. *Starting and Managing Your Practice: A Guide Book for Physicians.* Oelgeschlager, 1983.

Cuadca-Elsewar Staff. *Online Databases in the Medical and Life Sciences.* Elsevier, 1987.

Davis, James E., ed. *Major Ambulatory Surgery.* Williams and Wilkins, 1986.

Eiseman, Ben. *Cost-Effective Surgical Management* (Illus.). Saunders, 1987.

Gillette, R.D., *Procedures in Ambulatory Care.* McGraw, 1987.

Goldberg, Alvin, and Pegels, C. Carl. *Quality Circles in Health Care Facilities.* Aspen Pub., 1984.

Goldfield, Norbert, and Goldsmith, Seth B. *Financial Management of Ambulatory Care.* Aspen Pub., 1984.

Physician's Office and Ambulatory Surgery: Detailed Survey Data of Value to Medical, Insurance and High Tech Industries, FIND SVP., 1986.

Quality Assurance in Ambulatory Health Care. Joint Comm. Hosp., 1987.

Rostenberg, Bill. *Design Planning for Freestanding Ambulatory Care Facilities: A Primer for Health Care Providers and Architects.* AHPI, 1987.

Snook, I. Donald, and Kaye, Edita M. *A Guide to Health Care Joint Ventures*. Aspen Pub., 1986.

Sokin, Alan. *Health Care and the Changing Economic Environment*. Lexington Bks., 1985.

Wetchler, Bernard. *Anesthesia for Ambulatory Surgery*. Lippincott, 1985.

Chapter 6

Batalden, Paul B., and O'Conner, J. Paul. *Quality Assurance in Ambulatory Care*. Aspen Pub., 1980.

Dooley, Tricia C. *Ambulatory Care: Subject Index and Research Bibliography*. ABBE Pubs Assn., 1987.

Ellis, David. *Medical Computing and Applications*. Halsted Pr., 1987.

Gardocki, Gloria J. *Utilization of Outpatient Care Resources,* Cox, Klaudia, ed. Natl. Ctr. Health Stats., 1983.

Gardocki, Gloria J., et al. *The National Ambulatory Medical Care Complement Survey: United States, 1980*. Natl. Ctr. Health Stats., 1984.

Knutson, Karen, et al. *Ambulatory Care Nursing Standards and Performance Evaluations,* Center for Research in Ambulatory Health Care, Administration Staff, ed. Ctr. Res. Ambulatory.

O.R. Product Directory, 2nd Ed., 1989. Association of Operating Room Nurses, Inc.

Reichertz, P.L., and Engelbrecht, R., eds. *Present Status of Computer Support in Ambulatory Care*. Springer-Verlag, 1987.

Ross, Austin, et al. *Ambulatory Care: Organization and Management*. Wiley, 1983.

Winston, William J., ed. *Marketing Ambulatory Care Services*. Haworth Press, 1985.

Chapter 7

Bassett, L.W., et al. *Breast Cancer Detection: One Versus Two Views*. Radiology 165: 95-97, 1987.

Brenner, R.J. *Medical-Legal Aspects of a Screening Mammography: A Primer*. American Roentgen Ray Society Categorical Course Syllabus on Breast Imaging 1988: 121-128.

Carpman, Janet R., et al. *Design That Cares: Planning Health Facilities for Patients and Visitors*. AHPI, 1986.

Feig, S.A. *Screen-Film Mammography: Equipment, Technique, Quality Control*. American Roentgen Ray Society Categorical Course Syllabus on Breast Imaging 1988: 9-26.

Gold, R.H., et al. *Mammography Screening: Successes and Problems in Implementing Widespread Use in the United States.* Radiological Clinics of North America 25: no. 5: 1039-1046, September, 1987.

Hospital Economics and Medical Services: Subject Analysis Index With Reference Bibliography. ABBE Pubs Assn., 1987.

Howard, J. *Using Mammography for Cancer Control: An Unrealized Potential.* CA - A Cancer Journal for Clinicians 37: no. 1: 33-48, January/February 1987.

Koebetz, Wilson R. *Mammography in Health and Medicine: Research Subject Analysis with Reference Bibliography.* ABBE Pubs Assn., 1987.

Margolin, F.R., and Lagios, M.D. *Development of Mammography and Breast Services in a Community Hospital.* Radiologic Clinics of North America 25: no. 5: 973-982, September, 1987.

McLelland, R. *How to Establish a Low-Cost Community Screening Program for Breast Cancer.* American Roentgen Ray Society Categorical Course Syllabus on Breast Imaging 1988: 113-116.

Monsees, B., et al. *The Self-Referred Mammography Patient: A New Responsibility for Radiologists.* Radiology 166: 69-70, 1988.

Moskowitz, M. *Issues in Screening.* American Roentgen Ray Society Categorical Course Syllabus on Breast Imaging 1988: 105-112.

Quarles, Lucille W., *Attitudes of Consumers to Health and Care: Medical Analysis Index with Reference Bibliography.* ABBE Pubs Assn., 1987.

Russell, Louise B. *Is Prevention Better than Cure?* Brookings, 1986.

Sickles, E.A. *Impact of Low-Cost Mammography Screening on Nearby Mammography Practices.* Radiology 168: 59-61, 1988.

Tabar, L., and Dean, P.B. *The Control of Breast Cancer Through Mammography Screening.* Radiologic Clinics of North America 25: no. 5: 993-1005, September 1987.

Walsh, Charles H., and Walker, Morton. *Medical Practice Management Desk Book.* Prentice Hall, 1982.

Chapter 8

Birnbaum, Howard, et al. *Public Pricing of Nursing Home Care* (Illus.). U Pr of Amer., 1984.

Clarke, Freda. *Hospital at Home: The Alternative to General Hospital Admission.* Macmillan Ed UK, 1984.

Cooney, Cyprian J. *The Awakening of the Nursing Home Industry.* C C Thomas, 1986.

Debella, Sandra. *Nurse's Role in Health Care Planning.* Appleton and Lange, 1986.

Ensher, Gail L., and Clark, David A. *Newborns at Risk: Medical Care and Psychoeducational Intervention.* Aspen Pub., 1986.

Feller, Barbara A. *Americans Needing Home Care: United States.* USGPO, 1986.

Health Care at Home: An Essential Component of National Health Policy, Ch-9, ANA, 1978.

Health Care Cost Management. Intl. Found. Employ., 1986.

Health Care Cost Management-1985. Intl. Found. Employ., 1986.

Home-Based Chronic Care Markets, 1985-1990. Market Res Co.

Johnson, Everett A., and Johnson, Richard L. *Hospitals Under Fire.* Aspen Pub., 1986.

Lerman, Dan, ed. *Home Care: Positioning the Hospital for the Future.* AHPI, 1987.

McDonnell, Alice. *Quality Hospice Care: Administration, Organization, and Models.* Pub. by Natl Health Pub., Rynd Comm., 1985.

Miller, Susan C. *Documentation for Home Health Care: A Record Management Hand-book.* Am Med Record Assn., 1986.

Chapter 9

Blecke, C. *Patient Education. Home Chemotherapy Safety Procedures.* Oncol-Nurs-Forum, Sept.-Oct., 1989.

Butler, M.C. *Families' Responses to Chemotherapy by an Ambulatory Infusion Pump.* Nurs-Clin-North-Am., Mar., 1984.

Christ, G., and Siegel, K. *Monitoring Quality-of-Life Needs of Cancer Patients.* Cancer, Feb. 1, 1990.

Doyle, Derek, ed. *Palliative Care: The Management of Far Advanced Illness.* Charles, 1984.

Esparza, D.M., Young, N., and Luongo, J.A. *Effective Planning for Office and Outpatient Chemotherapy Administration.* Semin-Oncol-Nurs., May 1989.

Joseph, R., Dolby, P., and Forrest, J. *Home Chemotherapy: Problems, Pitfalls, Considerations, and Solutions.* Prog-Clin-Biol-Res., 1986.

Journal of Intravenous Nursing. Vol. 11, No. 1; Jan./Feb. 1988. J.B. Lippincott Company.

Lantz, James E. *An Introduction to Clinical Social Work Practice* (Illus.). C C Thomas, 1987.

Mor, V., Stalker, M.Z., Gralla, R., Scher, H.I., Cimma, C., Park, D., Flaherty, A.M., Kiss, M., Nelson, P., Laliberte, L., et al. *Day Hospital as an Alternative to Inpatient Care for Cancer Patients: A Random Assignment Trial.* J-Clin-Epidemiol, 1988.

Reville, B., and Almadrones, L. *Continuous Infusion Chemotherapy in the Ambulatory Setting: The Nurse's Role in Patient Selection and Education.* Oncol-Nurs-Forum, July-Aug., 1989.

Sansivero, G.E., and Murray, S.A. *Patient Education. Safe Management of Chemotherapy at Home.* Oncol-Nurs-Forum, Sept.-Oct., 1989.

Stevens, K.R. *Safe Handling of Cytotoxic Drugs in Home Chemotherapy.* Semin-Oncol-Nurs, May 1989.

Vinciguerra, V., Degnan, T.J., Budman, D.R., Brody, R.S., Moore, T., Sciortino, A., O'Connell, M. *Comparative Cost Analysis of Home and Hospital Treatment.* Prog-Clin-Biol-Res., 1986.

Vinciguerra, V., Degnan, T.J., Sciortino, A., O'Connell, M., Moore, T., Brody, R., Budman, D., Eng, M., Carlton, D. *A Comparative Assessment of Home Versus Hospital Comprehensive Treatment for Advanced Cancer Patients.* J-Clin-Oncol., Oct. 1986.

Vokes, E.E., Schilsky, R.L., Choi, K.E., Magid, D.M., Guarnieri, C.M., Whaling, S.M., Ratain, M.J., Weichselbaum, R.R., and Pahje, W.R. *A Randomized Study of Inpatient Versus Outpatient Continuous Infusion Chemotherapy for Patients with Locally Advanced Head and Neck Cancer.* Cancer, Jan. 1, 1989.

Wentzel, Kenneth B. *To Those Who Need It Most, Hospice Means Hope.* Charles River Bks., 1980.

Wohl, Stanley, and Schiff, Isaac. *Extended Patient Care: A Guide for Nursing Facilities.* InfoMed Bks., 1986.

Chapter 10

Bassett, Lawrence, and Metzger, Norman. *Achieving Excellence: A Prescription for Health Care Managers.* Aspen Pub., 1986.

Burrows, Seymour J. *Win-Win Outcomes: A Physician's Negotiating Guide. Pluribus Pr., 1984.*

Jennett, Bryan. *High Technology Medicine: Benefits and Burdens.* Oxford U Pr., 1986.

Kaufmann, H.J., ed. *Medical Imaging, No. 1* (Illus.). S Karger, 1980.

Novelline and Squire. *Living Anatomy: A Workbook Using Computed Tomography, Magnetic Resonance and Angiography.* Mosby, 1986.

Young, Stuart W., Jr., and Bartrum, Royal J., Jr. *Financial Independence: The Doctor's Guide.* Raven, 1984.

Chapter 11

Allswang, John. *Physician's Guide to Computers and Computing.* Appleton and Lange, 1985.

Anderson, Odin, et al. *HMOs Development: Patterns and Prospects.* Pluribus Pr., 1985.

Brown, J.H. *The High Cost of Healing: Physicians and the Health Care System.* Human Sci. Pr., 1985.

Center for Research in Ambulatory Health Care Administration Staff. *Evaluating the Performance of the Prepaid Medical Group: A Management Audit Manual.* Ctr Res Ambulatory, 1985.

Ginzberg, Eli. *From Physician Shortage to Patient Shortage: The Uncertain Future of Medical Practice.* Westview, 1986.

Ginzberg, Eli, and Ostow, Miriam. *The Coming Physician Surplus: In Search of a Public Policy.* Rowman, 1984.

Harris, John M. *The Role of the Medical Director in the Fee-for-Service Prepaid Medical Group.* Ctr Res Ambulatory, 1983.

Latham, W. Bryan. *Management of Medical Cost.* AMACOM, 1986.

MacFarlane, Peter W. *Computer Techniques in Clinical Medicine* (Illus.). Butterworth, 1986.

Professional Practice in Health Care Marketing: Proceedings of American College of Healthcare Marketing. (Health Marketing Quarterly Ser.: Vol. 3). Haworth Pr., 1986.

Scheffler, Richard M., and Rossiter, Louis F., eds. *Advances in Health Economics and Health Services Research: Mergers in Health Care - The Performance of Multi-Institutional Organizations,* Vol. 7, Jai Pr., 1986.

Schwefel, D., ed. *Indicators and Trends in Health and Health Care* (Illus.). Springer-Verlag, 1986.

Shaffer, Franklin A., ed. *Patients and Purse Strings: Patient Classification and Cost Management.* Natl League Nurse., 1986.

Sheldon, Alan, and Windham, Susan R. *Competitive Strategy for Health Care Organizations.* Dow Jones-Irwin, 1984.

Smith, Gilbert, and Cantly, Caroline. *Assessing Health Care: A Study in Organizational Evaluation.* Taylor and Francis, 1985.

Winston, William J. *How to Write a Marketing Plan for Health Care Organizations,* (Health Marketing Quarterly Supplement Ser.: Vol. 2). Haworth Pr., 1985.

Winston, William J., ed. *Health Marketing and Consumer Behavior: A Guide to Basic Linkages,* (Health Marketing Quarterly Ser.: Vol. 3, No. 1), Haworth Pr., 1985.

Zimmerman, David H. *Twelve Strategies to Improve Cash Flow in Medical Groups.* Ctr Res Ambulatory, 1985.

Chapter 12

Aaron, Henry J., and Schwartz, William B. *The Painful Prescription: Rationing Hospital Care.* Brookings, 1984.

Allen, James E. *Nursing Home Administration.* Springer Pub., 1987.

Betson, Carol L. *Managing the Medical Enterprise: A Study of Physician Managers.* UMI Res Pr., 1986.

Blanken, Gary E. *Surgical Operations in Short-Stay Hospitals, U.S. 1971.* Natl Ctr Health Stats., 1974.

Coile, Russell C., Jr. *The New Hospital: Future Strategies for a Changing Industry.* Aspen Pub., 1985.

Elrod, James L., Jr., et al. *Merging Care Institutions: A Guidebook for Buyers and Sellers.* AHPI, 1987.

Fagerhaugh, Shizuko Y., et al. *Hazards in Hospital Care: Ensuring Patient Safety.* Jossey-Bass, 1987.

Flynn, George. *Medicine in the Age of the Computer.* Prentice Hall, 1986.

Gardocki, Gloria J., and Pokras, Robert. *Utilization of Short-Stay Hospitals by Persons with Heart Disease and Malignant Neoplasms.* Natl Ctr Health Stats, 1981.

Griffith, John R. *The Well-Managed Community Hospital.* Health Admin Pr., 1987.

Hamill, Charlotte M. *The Day Hospital: Organization and Management.* Springer Pub., 1981.

Hass-Unger, Joan. *How to Survive in the Hospital.* Fischer Pub., 1986.

Martin, John P. *Hospitals in Trouble.* Basil Blackwell, 1985.

McMillan, Norman H., and Rosenbaum, George. *Managing Smart: Market Research for Hospital Decision Makers.* AHPI, 1986.

Meshenberg, Kathryn A., and Burns, Linda A., eds. *Hospital Ambulatory Care: Making It Work.* AHPI, 1983.

Nackel, John G., and Kis, George M. *Cost Management for Hospitals.* Aspen Pub., 1987.

Nich, David L., and Barrett, Michael J. *Effective Health Care Internal Auditing.* Aspen Pub., 1985.

Pokras, Robert. *Detailed Diagnosis and Procedures for Patients Discharged from Short-Stay Hospitals: United States, 1985.* USGPO, 1987.

Smith, Howard L., and Reid, Richard A. *Competitive Hospitals: Management Strategies.* Aspen Pub., 1986.

Stevens, Peter J., and McCleary, Ken W., eds. *The Marketing of Hospitality Services: Current Issues and Perspectives.* Hosp Pubns, 1986.

Sullivan, Catherine F. *Management of Medical Foodservice* (Illus.). AVI, 1985.

Chapter 13

Danzon, Patricia M. *Medical Malpractice: Theory, Evidence and Public Policy* (Illus.). Harvard U Pr., 1985.

Huston, Phillips. *Insurance Strategies for Physicians*. Med Economics, 1983.

King, Mark, et al. *Irresistible Communication: Creative Skills for the Health Professional* (Illus.). Saunders, 1983.

Lewis, Scott M., and McCutchen, Jeffrey R. *Emergency Medical Malpractice*. Wiley, 1987.

Major Health Issues for State Legislatures. Natl Conf State Legis., 1985.

McCafferty, Michael D., and Meyer, Steven M. *Medical Malpractice: Bases of Liability*. Shepards-McGraw, 1985.

Sarner, Harvey, and Lassiter, Herbert C. *Insurance for the Doctor*. Bks Demand UMI.

Shandell, Richard E. *The Preparation and Trial of Medical Malpractice Cases*. NY Law Pub., 1985.

Tobias, Andrew. *Treating Malpractice: Report of the Twentieth Century Fund Task Force on Medical Malpractice Insurance*. Priority Pr Pubns., 1986.

Zimmerman, Roy R. *Malpractice II: Legislation and Jurisprudence with Subject Analysis and Bibliography*. ABBE Pubs Assn., 1985.

Chapter 14

Barger, et al. *The PPO Handbook*. Aspen Pub., 1984.

Blank, Robert H. *Rationing Medicine* (Illus.). Columbia U Pr., 1988.

Blum, John, and Gertman, Paul M. *PSROs and the Law*. Aspen Pub., 1977.

Bonham, Gordon S. *Content and Instruments of the National Medical Care Utilization and Expenditure Survey,* Michael, Geraldine, ed. Natl. Ctr. Health Stats., 1982.

Brown, J.H. *Management in Health Care Systems*. CRC Pr., 1984.

Coddington, Dean C., and Moore, Keith D. *Market Driven Strategies in Health Care*. Jossey Bass, 1987.

Cooper, Philip D. *Health Care Marketing: Issues and Trends,* 2nd ed. Aspen Pub., 1985.

Cooper, Philip D., ed. *Responding to the Challenge: Health Care Marketing Comes of Age*. Am Mktg., 1986.

Cowan, Dale H. *Preferred Provider Organizations: Planning, Structure and Operation.* Aspen Pub., 1984.

Fox, Peter D., and Heinen, LuAnn. *Determinants of HMO Success.* Health Admin Pr., 1987.

Ginzberg, Eli. *From Physician Shortage to Patient Shortage: The Uncertain Future of Medical Practice.* Westview, 1986.

Goldfield, Norbert, and Goldsmith, Seth B. *Alternative Delivery Systems.* Aspen Pub., 1986.

Kurowski, Bettina D., ed. *Meeting the Healthcare Needs of Business: A Guide for Medical Groups.* Med Group Mgmt.

Leutz, Walter N., et al. *Changing Health Care for an Aging Society: Planning for the Social Health Maintenance Organization.* Lexington Bks., 1985.

Mackie, Dustin, and Decker, Douglas. *Group and IPA HMOs.* Aspen Pub., 1981.

MacStravic, Robin D. *Managing Health Care Marketing Communications.* Aspen Pub., 1985.

McArdle, Frank B., ed. *The Changing Health Care Market.* U Pr of Amer., 1987.

Medicare and Prepaid Health Plans: New Directions for HMOs. AMA, 1985.

Physician's Guide to Preferred Provider Organizations. AMA, 1984.

QRB Special Edition: Data Management in Cost Containment and Quality Review Strategies. Joint Comm Hosp., 1983.

Skuby, Eugenia W., and White, Elizabeth H., eds. *HMO Physician Managers Managing HMO Physicians.* Group Health Assoc of Amer., 1985.

Snider, Erica M. *Health Maintenance Organizations: Subject Analysis with Reference Bibliography.* ABBE Pubs Assn., 1987.

Tibbits, Samuel J., and Manzano, Allen J. *PPOs: An Executive's Guide.* Pluribus Pr, 1984.

Wagner, Eric R., and Hackenberg, Valerie J. *A Practical Guide to Physician-Sponsored HMO Development.* Am Soc Intern Med., 1986.

Wolfson, Jay, and Levin, Peter J. *Managing Employee Health Benefits: A Guide to Cost Control.* Dow Jones-Irwin, 1985.

Yaggy, Duncan, and Hodgson, Patricia, eds. *How Many Doctors Do We Need? (A Policy Agenda for the U.S. in the 1990s Based on the Tenth Private Sector Conference, 1985).* Duke, 1986.

Chapter 15

Graves, Edmund J. *Inpatient Utilization of Short-Stay Hospitals by Diagnosis, United States: PHS 87-1750,* Cox, Klaudia, Ed. Natl Ctr Health Stats., 1987.

Levine, Marshall R. *A Physician's Guide to Utilization Review.* Davis Co., 1986.

Minckley, Barbara B., and Walters, Mary D., eds. *Health Care Cost Containment: Dilemmas and Solutions.* Midwest Alliance Nursing, 1984.

Pletcher, Suzette M. *Health Care Cost Containment: Strategies That Work for You, Your Employees, and Your Company.* Busn. Legal Reports, 1986.

Skillicorn, Stanley A. *Ensuring Quality in an Era of Cost Containment* (Illus.). Am. Health Consults, 1986.

Tourangeau, Roger, and Rasinski, Kenneth A. *Evaluation of Data Collection Frequency and the Data Summary in the National Medical Care Utilization and Expenditure Survey, PHS.* Olmsted, Mary, ed. Natl Ctr Health Stats., 1987.

Chapter 16

Berry, F.A., M.D. *Pre-Operative Assessment and General Management of Outpatients.* International Anesthesiology Clinics, 20(1), 1982.

Boroson, Warren. *Physician's Guide to Professional and Personal Advisers.* Med Economics, 1985.

Botello, Nina. *Material Management in Same Day Surgery.* FASA Update, May 1989.

Burns, Linda. *Ambulatory Surgery: Developing and Managing Successful Programs.* Aspen Publications, 1984.

Burns, Linda A., and Mancino, Douglas M. *Joint Ventures Between Hospitals and Physicians: A Competitive Strategy for the Healthcare Marketplace.* Dow Jones-Irwin, 1986.

Ernst and Whinney. *Procedural Cost Manual for Ambulatory Surgery Centers.* Federated Ambulatory Surgical Association, 1989.

Hardy, Owen B., and Lammers, Lawrence P. *Hospitals: The Planning and Design Process,* 2nd ed. Aspen Pub., 1986.

Healthcare Financial Management Assn. *Capital Management in Healthcare Organizations: Capital Investment and Financing Strategies* (Illus.). Healthcare Fin Mgmt Assn., 1984.

Lisbon, Alan, M.D. *Anesthetic Considerations in Setting Up a New Medical Facility.* International Anesthesiology Clinics, 19(2), 1981.

Nackel, John G., et al. *Working with Health Care Consultants* (Illus.). AHPI, 1986.

Natof, Herbert E., M.D. *Complications Associated with Ambulatory Surgery*. Journal of the American Medical Association, 244: 1116-1118, 1980.

Planning Guide for Physicians' Medical Facilities. AMA, 1986.

Scheyer, William L. *Handbook of Health Care Material Management*. Aspen Pub., 1985.

Standards for Ambulatory Health Care. Accreditation Association for Ambulatory Health Care. 1988.

U.S. Department of Health and Human Services. *Minimum Requirements of Construction and Equipment for Hospital and Medical Facilities*. USGPO, July 1984.

Wong, Harry, M.D. *General Anesthesia for Ambulatory Surgery*. International Anesthesiology Clinics, 20(1), 1982.

Ziegler, A. *Supplies and Office Maintenance,* Vol. 8. (Illus.). Med Economics, 1982.

Suggested Additional Reading

American Hospital Association. *Hospital Statistics: Data from the American Hospital Association 1986 Annual Survey,* (Illus.). Am Hospital, 1987.

Berman, Howard J., et al. *The Financial Management of Hospitals,* 6th ed. Health Admin Pr., 1986.

Directory of Multihospital Systems, 1985. Am Hospital, 1985.

Egdahl, Richard H., and Walsh, Diana C., eds. *Industry and Health Care, Vol. 2: Health Cost Management and Medical Practice Patterns.* Ballinger Pub., 1985.

Eisenberg, John M. *Doctors' Decisions and the Cost of Medical Care: The Reasons for Doctors' Practice Patterns and Ways to Change Them.* Health Admin Pr., 1986.

Fallek, Max. *How to Set Up and Operate Your Own Health Care Practice.* Amer Inst Small Bus., 1987.

Garg, Mohan L., and Kleinberg, Warren M. *Clinical Training and Health Care Costs: A Basic Curriculum for Medical Education.* Praeger, 1985.

Ginsberg, Stephen P. *The Out-Patient Ophthalmic Surgery Center.* Slack Inc., 1985.

Goldstone, L.A. *Understanding Medical Statistics.* Heinman, 1984.

Grupenhoff, John T. *National Health Directory.* Aspen Pub., 1986.

Haberek, Judy. *One Hundred Twenty-Five Ways to Cut Your Business Health Costs,* Varela, Robert, ed. Wash. Busn. Info., 1985.

Health Care Financing Extramural Report: Evaluation of Community-Oriented Long-Term Care Demonstration Projects. USGPO, 1987.

Healthcare Online, Vol. 1, No. 1, Oct. 1985. Medical Data Exchange Inc.

Hillestad, Steven G., and Berkowitz, Eric W. *Health Care Marketing Plans: From Strategy to Action.* Dow Jones-Irwin, 1984.

Hospital Strategy Report, Vol. 1, No. 1 (Nov. 1988). Aspen Systems Corporation.

Hughes, Susan. *Long Term Care: Options in an Expanding Market.* Dow Jones-Irwin, 1986.

Inlander, Charles B., and Weiner, Ed. *Take This Book to the Hospital with You: A Consumer's Guide to Surviving Your Hospital Stay.* Warner Bks., 1987.

Jacobs, Philip. *The Economics of Health and Medical Care,* 2nd ed. Aspen Pub., 1986.

Jaeger, B. Jon, et al., eds. *Multi-Instructional Systems Management: Concepts and Cases.* AUPHA Pr., 1987.

Jonas, Steven. *Health Care Delivery in the United States,* 3rd ed. Springer Pub., 1986.

Jones, Rochelle. *The Supermeds: How Private For-Profit Medical Conglomerates Are Controlling Our Health Care and What We Can Do About It.* Scribners, 1987.

Joseph, Eric D., et al. *Physician Practice Monitors.* Care Comm Inc., 1986.

King, Martha P. *What Legislators Need to Know About Health Data-Cost Information Programs.* Natl. Conf. State Legis., 1986.

Kruzas, Anthony T., et al., eds. *Encyclopedia of Medical Organizations and Agencies,* 2nd ed. Gale, 1986.

Kruzas, Anthony T., et al. *Medical and Health Information Directory,* Vol. 3, 3rd ed. Gale, 1986.

Luke, Roice D., and Krueger, Janelle. *Organization and Change in Health Care Quality Assurance.* Aspen Pub., 1983.

Market Intelligence Research Company Staff. *Disposable Medical Products,* Hammersley, W., ed. Market Res Co., 1986.

McMahon, Carol E. *Where Medicine Fails.* Trado-Medic, 1986.

Mooney, Gavin. *Economics, Medicine and Health Care,* (Illus.). Humanities, 1986.

Moore, Terence F., and Simendinger, Earl A. *The Effective Health Care Executive.* Aspen Pub., 1986.

Multihospital Systems: Perspective and Trends. Am Hospital, 1987.

Nursing Home Industry. Busn. Trend, 1986.

O'Brien, Jacqueline Wasserman, and Wasserman, Steven R., eds. *Statistics Sources, Thirteenth Edition, 1990.* Gale Research Inc., 1990.

Orlikoff, James E., and Snow, Anita. *Assessing Quality Circles in Health Care Settings: A Guide for Management.* AHPI, 1984.

Paul, D. Terry, ed. *Building Marketing Effectiveness in HealthCare.* Am Mktg, 1985.

Pennsylvania Bar Institute. *Joint Ventures in Health Care.* PA Bar Inst., 1985.

Physician's Guide to Professional Corporations. AMA, 1984

Physician's Resource Guide to Health Delivery Systems. AMA, 1987.

Physician-Hospital Joint Ventures. AMA, 1986.

Planning Guide for Physicians' Medical Facilities. AMA, 1986.

Rahn, Gary J., ed. *Hospital-Sponsored Health Maintenance Organizations: Issues for Decision Makers.* AHPI, 1987.

Rice, James A., II, and Creel, George H. *Market-Based Demand Forecasting for Hospital Inpatient Services.* AHPI, 1985.

Robin, Eugene D. *Medical Care Can Be Dangerous to Your Health: A Guide to the Risks and Benefits.* Har-Row, 1986.

Rosenberg, Charles E. *The Care of Strangers: The Rise of America's Hospital System.* Basic, 1987.

Rubel, Arthur J., et al. *Susto: A Folk Illness,* Leslie, Charles, ed. (Illus.). U of Cal. Pr., 1985.

Saari, Carolyn. *Clinical Social Work Treatment: How Does It Work?* Gardner Pr., 1986.

Scheffler, Richard. *Advances in Health Economics and Health Services Research,* Vol. 6. Jai Pr, 1986.

Schwartz, Ronald M., et al, eds. *Group Health, 1986: Institute Proceedings, New Health Care Systems: HMOs and Beyond.* Group Health Assoc. of Amer., 1987.

Smith, David B., and Kaluzny, Arnold D. *The White Labyrinth: A Guide to the Health Care System,* 2nd ed. Health Admin Pr., 1986.

Smith, Howard L., and Elbert, Norbett. *The Health Care Supervisor's Guide to Staff Development.* Aspen Pub., 1985.

Sunshine, Linda, and Wright, John W. *The Best Hospitals in America.* H. Holt and Co., 1987.

Troyer, Glen T., and Salman, Steven I. *Handbook of Health Care Risk Management.* Aspen Pub., 1985.

Virgo, John M., ed. *Exploring New Vistas in Health Care.* IHEMI, 1985.

West, Ruth, and Trevelyn, Joanna. *Alternative Medicine: A Bibliography of Books in English.* Mansell, 1985.

Williamson, John W., et al. *Principles of Quality Assurance and Cost Containment in Health Care: A Guide for Medical Students, Residents and Other Health Professionals.* Jossey Bass, 1982.

Yanda, Roman L. *Doctors as Managers of Health Teams: A Career Guide for Hospital-Based Physicians.* Bks Demand UMI.

Young, David W., and Saltman, Richard B. *The Hospital Power Equilibrium: Physician Behavior and Cost Control.* Johns Hopkins, 1985.

Zimmerman, Roy R. *Quality of Health Care Research Reference Analysis with Bibliography.* ABBE Pubs. Assn., 1987.